How To Lower Blood Sugar

Natural Remedies for Diabetes

Nora M. Greenway

© 2012 by Nora M. Greenway and Creative Bookworm Press

ISBN-13:   978-0-9791653-3-7
ISBN-10:   0-9791653-3-4

This publication is designed to provide accurate and authoritative educational information in regard to the subject matter covered. It is sold with the understanding that the author/publisher is not engaged in rendering medical, health, dietary, nutritional, legal, accounting, or other professional services or individualized professional advice. If medical advice or other expert assistance is required, the services of a competent professional person should be sought.

First Printing, 2012

Printed in the United States of America

Creative Bookworm Press, Tucson AZ USA

Liability Disclaimer

The information provided here offers an educational resource only and is not intended to serve as specific or individualized nutritional, dietary, health, or medical advice related to any person's diet or health problems. There can be no assurance that any person's specific diet or health problems, diseases, or symptoms will heal, recover, or otherwise resolve as a result of applying the information provided here or in other resources mentioned in the book.

There also can be no assurance of safety with or absence of possible harm from any specific strategy, treatment or therapy if a specific person tries such treatment or therapy mentioned in this book, or other media. The reader is advised to seek personalized advice from a qualified health care provider, nutritionist, and/or dietician before attempting to implement information provided in this book.

Neither the author nor the publisher assumes any responsibility for any errors or omissions. The author and publisher also specifically disclaim any responsibility or liability resulting from the use of any of the information discussed in this book.

Terms of Use

This is copyrighted material. Your purchase of this book gives you a non-transferable, "personal use" license. You do not have any resale rights or private label rights from this book purchase.

How To Lower Blood Sugar

Natural Remedies for Diabetes

Table of Contents

What Is Diabetes?

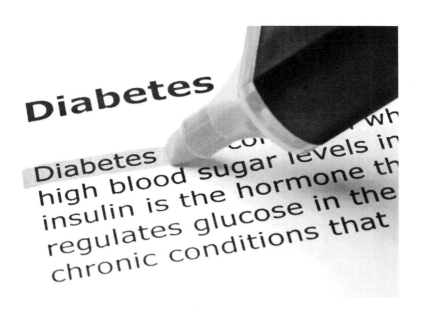

Diabetes mellitus (DM) is a metabolic disorder that affects millions of adults and children. DM is a leading cause of death and disability in the United States.

The statistics are distressing -- over 79 million adults and children have prediabetes (and many do not even realize it), and 25.8 million adults and children have full-blown diabetes in the United States alone. Diabetes costs the U.S. over $174 billion per year. In a period of tough economic times, this is an incredibly costly condition, with a severe impact on the lives and finances of patients, their families, and society overall.

If you have diabetes, the glucose (sugar) levels in your blood get too high. The basic problem in diabetes is that the cells in your body cannot use sugar in the blood stream normally. When this happens, the excess sugar damages many different parts of your body in the short- and long-term. High blood sugar levels can wreak havoc with your heart, blood vessels, kidneys, and nerves. Diabetics often have problems healing from seemingly minor injuries.

The eventual serious risks are increased rates of heart attacks, strokes, kidney failures, loss of vision, amputations of limbs, and excruciating pain in the feet and hands.

The good news is that with proper lifestyle changes and treatment, it is possible to drastically improve your odds of a healthier and longer life. But this is a disorder in which you cannot be the spectator. You have to become an active participant and take charge of your own health and health care on a day-to-day basis. This book focuses on the natural ways to lower blood sugar and protect your body from diabetic complications.

Let's take a closer look at the specifics.

In the course of digesting food, your body breaks down what you eat into fuel to run your cells. The main fuel that results from metabolism is a simple sugar called glucose. You can make glucose from carbohydrates, proteins, or fats in food, but it is carbohydrates that break down into the largest amount of glucose and raise your blood sugar level the fastest. Research also shows that diets high in fat, calories, and cholesterol tend to raise your risk of developing diabetes.

One way or another, in diabetes, you have a problem with the hormone that regulates glucose in your body, insulin. There are two common reasons for the high blood glucose levels in diabetes -- either (1) your pancreas, the digestive gland that makes and secretes insulin, can no longer generate this hormone at all (Type 1); or (2) the cells of your body fail to respond to the insulin that your pancreas sends out to do its job, i.e., insulin resistance (Type 2).

Type 1 diabetes represents 5-10% of the condition. It is an autoimmune disorder in which the body attacks its own cells in the pancreas (beta cells) that make insulin, destroying them. This leaves the person dependent on daily insulin injections to stay alive. Although Type 1 can develop at any age, the most common time is in childhood or early adulthood.

Experts are not sure why type 1 diabetes autoimmunity happens, but it may involve exposure to certain viruses, gluten intolerance, genetics, toxins, vitamin D deficiency, and/or other environmental factors. Type 1 appears to be more common in whites than in nonwhites.

Type 2 diabetes is the most common form. Most people with this condition are older, and many are overweight. Type 2 diabetes often goes along with other health problems, including high blood pressure and high cholesterol. Risk factors for getting type 2 include obesity, family history of diabetes, and physical inactivity. Women with polycystic ovary syndrome have an increased risk of type 2 diabetes. Some drugs increase the risk of developing type 2 diabetes, including certain psychiatric and high blood pressure medications.

With the rise of obesity in young people, type 2 diabetes is becoming more common at much younger ages than used to be the case. People of all races and ethnicities can get diabetes, but there are higher rates in people who are African-American, Hispanic, Asian, and Native American.

There is a third type, called gestational diabetes, which only occurs in 3-8% of pregnant women and usually goes away after the baby is born. Gestational diabetes can be dangerous for both mother and baby, however. It is often a warning that the mother might go on to develop type 2 diabetes. Between 40 and 60% of women with gestational diabetes get type 2 diabetes within the next 5-10 years.

People with type 2 diabetes can develop the condition over a long period of time. If your blood sugar levels are increased, but not so high as to receive a diagnosis of diabetes, you may have a condition called prediabetes. Prediabetes is a warning to get started on taking steps to get your blood sugar under control – or face progression into a full case of diabetes, with its myriad of complications and treatment challenges.

Symptoms of Diabetes

The abnormalities of metabolism involved in diabetes cause a cascade of events leading to symptoms. The first step toward getting control of your blood sugar is arming yourself with some basic facts about diabetes. These will help you understand why certain types of natural treatments and remedies might help you lower high blood sugar levels and avoid, or at least delay the onset of diabetic complications.

The symptoms of high blood sugar or "hyperglycemia" include:

- frequent urination
- increased thirst
- fatigue or sleepiness
- headaches
- difficulty concentrating
- blurry vision
- unexplained weight loss even if appetite is normal
- skipped or absent menstrual periods in teen girls and women

People with high blood sugar, including "prediabetes," can have these same symptoms, even without a full diagnosis of diabetes. Still, some people with prediabetes and diabetes do not notice any symptoms at all. As a result, getting a screening test for blood sugar problems is very important if you have any risk factors for developing diabetes mellitus.

You want to see you doctor if you are having these symptoms and don't know why, since there are many other causes that also require a medical professional to test and diagnose the problem.

Symptoms of high blood sugar include poor wound healing of cuts or sores and repeated infections such as vaginal yeast infections or skin infections and vision problems from an overgrowth of extra blood vessels in the eye. Diabetics may get cataracts in the eyes sooner than other people. Eventually long-term high blood sugar levels can damage the nerves to the feet and hands so badly that you experience severe constant tingling, numbness, and pain in feet and hands. At some point, you stop feeling pain the way you should – and minor cuts can lead to loss of limbs or even death.

Blood Sugar Tests and Charts

Your doctor can do simple blood tests to check your blood sugar levels for the diagnosis. Typically, an important time to test is first thing in the morning when you are fasting before breakfast. This tells the doctor if you body can get itself back to a normal blood sugar level overnight without having to process any food.

A more functional test of your ability to regulate blood sugar is called the glucose tolerance test (GTT). In that test, the doctor gets a fasting blood sample and then asks you to drink a special sweet drink containing a standard amount of glucose or dextrose. Then they take additional blood samples periodically for a couple of hours after you drink the sugar solution. The GTT shows how well your body can handle a load of glucose all at once.

Once you hear that you have prediabetes or diabetes, however, it is up to you to monitor your blood sugar levels daily with a home test kit or glucose monitor. These systems require you to prick your finger or arm to get a drop of blood that you then place on a special test strip. With just a little research, you can find ways to get a blood glucose monitor kit very cheaply or for free. Many of the manufacturers know that they make most of their money from selling you box after box of the one-time use, disposable test strips on which you place each drop of blood. As a result, you can often find coupons or deep discounts for buying the meter itself. Insurance companies also usually pay for both the meters and test strips.

For people on insulin, there are also more elaborate continuous glucose monitoring devices that involve disposable sensors placed just under the skin on your abdomen. The sensors sample blood sugar every 5 minutes or so round the clock and send back wireless signals through transmitters to receivers that record the data.

These devices can give you quick feedback on what your blood sugar is doing – is it trending up or down and how fast is it changing. This is a type of biofeedback instrument that can warn you if you are going too high or low in time for you to take corrective action. Overall, continuous glucose monitoring can help you control blood sugar and avoid extremes – the exhausting highs of too much blood sugar or the dangerous jittery fuzzy-headed lows of excess insulin effects.

The charts below tell you the range for normal and abnormal blood sugar levels. Compare the values that you get from the tests done in your doctor's office and the ones that you do at home. This is where you really come into the picture. You can always choose to make up the findings from your home tests to make your doctor proud. But the only person you are hurting if you do something like that is yourself. Big time.

The hard facts of diabetes are that even if you think you can "cheat" on your diet so that no one else around you knows what you are eating, your body knows – it does not lie. It (and you) will pay the price every time you "cheat," whether you admit it to yourself or not.

So, here is your reality check:

A blood sugar levels chart can show you at a glance where your current blood sugar puts you on the range of possible normal and abnormal values. Blood sugar levels can be high or low. Both are dangerous to your health in different ways. High blood sugar is called "hyperglycemia" and low blood sugar is called "hypoglycemia."

There are different circumstances when doctors measure your blood sugar. After an overnight fast when you have not eaten for 8-12 hours is a basic way, but then you also need to test blood sugar after eating, typically about 2 hours after eating, to see how high the blood sugar went. Finally, doctors may have you do a test called an oral glucose tolerance test in which they give you a standard sweet drink in the clinical laboratory and take several blood samples before and after to see how your body handles a standard amount of pure sugar intake.

Here are blood sugar levels charts from a U.S. Government website at the National Institutes of Health to help you put your own blood sugar levels into perspective.

FPG means fasting blood or plasma glucose levels:

Table 1. FPG test

Plasma Glucose Result (mg/dL)	Diagnosis
99 or below	Normal
100 to 125	Pre-diabetes (impaired fasting glucose)
126 or above	Diabetes*

*Confirmed by repeating the test on a different day.

Here are the oral glucose tolerance test values (OGTT):

16

Table 2. OGTT

2-Hour Plasma Glucose Result (mg/dL)	Diagnosis
139 and below	Normal
140 to 199	Pre-diabetes (impaired glucose tolerance)
200 and above	Diabetes*

*Confirmed by repeating the test on a different day.

For women who are pregnant, they have somewhat more detailed cut-offs for blood sugar levels:

Table 3. Gestational diabetes: Above-normal results for the OGTT*

When	Plasma Glucose Result (mg/dL)
Fasting	95 or higher
At 1 hour	180 or higher
At 2 hours	155 or higher
At 3 hours	140 or higher

Note: Some laboratories use other numbers for this test.

*These numbers are for a test using a drink with 100 grams of glucose.

(Source: http://diabetes.niddk.nih.gov/dm/pubs/diagnosis/)

Another important blood test to monitor your progress in controlling your blood sugar is the HbA1c. This test sums up how much glucose has been sticking to part of the hemoglobin in your blood during the past 3–4 months. Hemoglobin is a substance in the red blood cells that supplies oxygen to the cells of the body. It helps mark how much damage you may be doing to your cells with the diabetes over time and thus risk of complications.

17

Get an HbA1C test done twice a year. Normal values are less than 5.7%. Prediabetes values can range from 5.7 to 6.4%, and diabetes values begin at 6.4%. Good diabetes control happens at or below 7.0%.

Your Action Steps:

1. Ask your doctor to test and tell you the level of your current fasting blood sugar.

2. If your blood sugar is elevated, even a little, get yourself a home glucose monitoring kit from your local pharmacy or online.

- It will include a meter, test strips, and a lancet device with disposable lancets to prick your finger or arm for a tiny sample of blood to put on the test strip.

- The newest lancet devices and lancets are so quick and simple to use, it barely hurts to do these life-saving tests.

- Learn how to test yourself for blood sugar levels at home.

3. Keep a journal of what you eat and what your blood sugar levels are immediately upon awakening in the morning before breakfast, before each subsequent meal, and then 2 hours after each meal. Do this for a week.

- Think about what you have learned from monitoring your blood sugar. We'll use it in the rest of this book.

- Bring this record to your doctor and work with him or her to develop a good treatment plan.

"The willingness to accept responsibility for one's own life is the source from which self-respect springs."

- Joan Didion

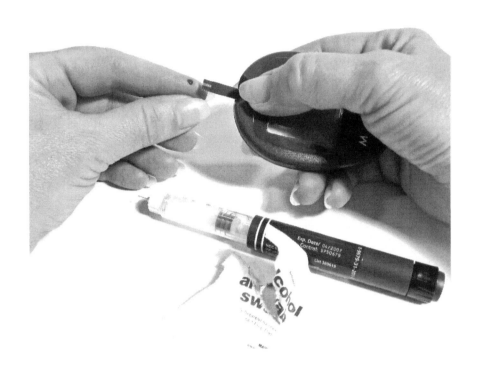

Low Carb Diet for Diabetes: Overview

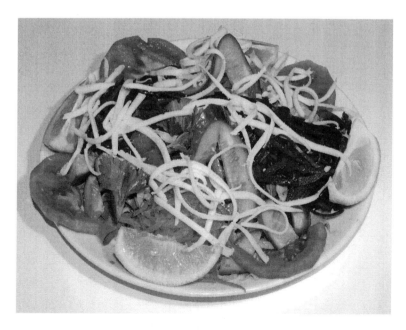

Balance is the key word in living well with diabetes. Strive for balance in all parts of your life, including your diet. With the support of your family and friends, your health care team, and your community, you can take charge of your diabetes.

Let's cut to the chase – the best diet plan for you if you have prediabetes or diabetes is a low carb (low in carbohydrates) diet.

Why? Even though eating sugar by itself is not necessarily the original cause of your diabetes, eating (or drinking) rapidly absorbed carbs, especially sugary sodas and foods and low fiber starches like white bread, will make your blood sugar soar.

You need to eat some amounts of carbohydrates, fats, and proteins for good health. Each "macronutrient" type brings in certain building blocks for a healthy body. What matters for your diet is choosing specific foods from each class of macronutrient that promote rather than tear down your health. We'll discuss the details of the right foods for you later in this book.

Major Diabetic Diet Principle 1:

Choose foods that work for you instead of against you.

Weight loss actually comes along for the ride if you stick with a good low carb diet plan. For example, if you just find a non-sugary alternative beverage to regular sodas, you can drop 10 pounds of fat per year! Not bad.

What are your alternatives for sodas? Try different beverages until you find ones that you like. Start with water, which is always a healthy, even essential, drink, and just make your own. Yes, you can even have homemade lemonade if you squeeze your own lemons into water and add stevia, a natural sweetener, instead of sugar. Also check out herb teas. Fruit flavored herb teas can taste sweet, and you can add stevia if you must have a sweeter taste.

Stevia is a no-calorie, no-brainer as a sweetener for diabetics. It is considered safe in amounts up to 4 milligrams per pound of body weight per day. If you weigh 150 pounds, you have lot of stevia to work with in a typical day (4 milligrams x 150 pounds = 600 mg/day).

In reality, stevia is so sweet, you'll find yourself satisfied with a drop or two of the liquid form or a packet of the powdered version of this sweetener (which contains just 80 mg of stevia per packet).

Also, herb teas containing hibiscus and those with anise or fennel may actually help you, respectively, control your blood pressure (hibiscus) and blood sugar (anise, fennel, with their sweet, licorice-like taste).

One word of caution -- Be careful to avoid herb teas that contain very much licorice per se - although this herb can have some beneficial effects in short-term use, it can raise your blood pressure a lot by causing your cells to hold onto sodium (salt).

Major Diabetic Diet Principle 2:

Replace refined starchy foods with high fiber and/or high protein versions of grains, pastas, and breads.

For example, if you become an avid label reader in the grocery store, you will find types of high fiber pastas that are not only whole wheat or brown rice-based, but also high in protein.

Foods high in fiber and/or high in protein tend to hit your blood stream more slowly than ordinary pastas like plain spaghetti or macaroni made from refined white flour.

What this means to you is less of a blood sugar peak after a pasta-containing meal when you do splurge with a side dish or main course of angel hair Italian food. Remember that your blood sugar goes up in the hours after you eat a meal or snack. How high it goes and how fast the blood sugar rises depends on what the food contains.

If you don't give your body a lot of carbs to deal with (and we know that it has a hard time processing carbs properly), your blood sugar level will be lower. It really is as simple as that.

Dealing with gluten intolerance? Many type 1 and type 2 diabetics may face this problem. Then try some of the products with alternative no-calorie, very low carb noodles (Shirataki), a traditional Japanese food made from natural water soluble fiber (see www.MiracleNoodle.com).

The lower the rise in blood sugar after a meal, the less you will need to take oral drugs like Metformin or injected insulin. The less drug you need, the fewer drug side effects you will experience. Since some diabetic drugs may even increase heart disease risk, the less you need to take, the better off you will be.

Of course, you have to take these drugs if you are not controlling your blood sugar adequately with diet, exercise, and natural remedies. Never decide to stop your medications suddenly. There are serious risks of not doing anything about your blood sugar. Still, if you have good options that can help you gradually reduce and maybe eliminate the need for drugs (with your doctor's supervision), this is a highly desirable way to go.

One of things that diabetics quickly discover is that these drugs do not have the safety stops in them that your body's own natural regulatory systems have. So, if you overtreat yourself with excess insulin, you risk a serious low blood sugar episode that can lead to loss of consciousness, confusion, behavioral changes, seizures, and even death. Some experts believe that having many serious low blood sugar episodes from excessive insulin treatment can promote long-term brain damage and dementia.

Your body has natural ways of counterbalancing the amounts and effects of insulin in the body – but it cannot regulate insulin injected from outside your body. You must use oral drugs and/or insulin if you insist on eating higher carb foods, but you can sidestep the problem by making wiser food choices.

This is not about depriving yourself of comfort foods. It's about you surviving and thriving. Even comfort foods come in healthier versions. Find them.

The Low Carb Diet Solution

The main bulk of low carb foods come from meats, non-starchy vegetables, nuts (raw or roasted, not sweetened or highly salted), salad vegetables and some fruits. Some low carb diabetic diets allow wholegrain bread and pasta to be eaten, but this will depend on the diet you choose.

Low carb recipes for diabetics can be found online as well as in recipe books. Once having come to grips with low carb eating you will soon find that many dishes can be adapted to low carb eating.

A low carb diabetic diet has been shown to address many of the problems associated with this disease and there are many low carb success stories to back this up and suggest that there are several low carb diets that work.

Again, it is important however, to remember that low carb does not mean no carb or a carb free diet. Deficiency of carbohydrates can in itself lead to health issues such as fatigue, impaired mental capacity and muscle cramps. Therefore you need to eat a certain number of carbohydrate grams per day.

What Are Carbohydrates?

Let's take a closer look at what carbohydrates are and how they work. You need to know a little basic chemistry first.

The function of carbs in your body is to provide the main source of energy for the body. Your body either uses the carbohydrates immediately or your body can convert them into fat to store and use later. Carbohydrates or saccharides are sugars and starches which provide energy for humans and animals. There are two types of carbohydrates, simple or monosaccharides and complex, or polysaccharides.

Simple carbohydrates are found in foods such as fruits and dairy and are more easily digested by the body. Because of the way our food is processed now, they are also often found in refined foods such as white sugar, pastas and white bread.

Complex carbohydrates on the other hand, take longer to digest and are mainly found in vegetables, whole grain breads and pastas, brown rice and legumes. The refining processes used today remove some of the grain's fiber and nutrients. Therefore, eating a bowl of whole grain cereal such as oatmeal (regular, not instant) will not only fill you up for longer but give you longer lasting energy than a bowl of sugary refined cereal due to the way the body uses and processes the carbohydrates in the food.

Once you have eaten carbs in food, it is the job of the liver to digest carbs by breaking them down into simple sugars or glucose. This in turn stimulates the production of insulin in the pancreas. The function of insulin is to convert this sugar into energy by getting it into the body's blood cells. Simple and complex carbohydrates affect the production of insulin in different ways.

As we have discussed, when digesting simple carbohydrates, insulin levels rise faster and 'spike' faster and the carbs are used up faster for energy. This is why when you eat a sugary sweet or snack to quickly satisfy hunger or for a quick energy burst, you find that energy levels crash soon after when the sugar 'high' ends. Complex carbohydrates take longer to digest.

This results in a longer lasting period of energy and -- importantly – a lower peak blood sugar level and less need for insulin to process the meal. Since the body of a diabetic does not release and/or use insulin well, needing less in the first place is a good thing.

If the body produces too much glucose, it will be stored in the liver and the muscle cells as glycogen. This is stored until the body next needs a burst of energy. Any glycogen that isn't stored in the liver or cells is stored in the body as fat. The body uses the immediate stores of glycogen for short term energy needs.

However, this is where the problem of being over-weight or developing diabetes can occur. If too much fat is stored and not used as energy, health problems may occur. Only when exercise or workouts are under-taken will your body use the reserves of fat as energy.

The recommended carbohydrate intake for an adult on a daily basis varies from one organization to another. The World Health Organization recommends 55-75% of dietary energy should come from carbohydrates. Only 10% should come from simple carbs. The Institute of Medicine recommends 40-65% from carbohydrates.

However, no one should have a carb free diet. The body needs a certain amount of carbs to function properly. If insufficient carbs are consumed it may result in health problems such as fatigue, poor mental capacity and muscle cramps. Your body will burn fat and even muscle to make the basic amounts of glucose it needs to run the body. Sure, that is a short term strategy for some fad diets, but it is not good for you in the long run. Eating a small amount of healthier carbs is the best plan.

Summary:

The body can produce energy from fat and proteins alone, making very low carb diets and the consumption of foods low in carbs possible. But, remember that low-carb does not mean totally no-carb. Eating the right types of carbs is important for dieting to get healthy weight loss and develop healthy eating habits over the long haul...that is, for a healthier happier life.

Glycemic Index and Glycemic Load

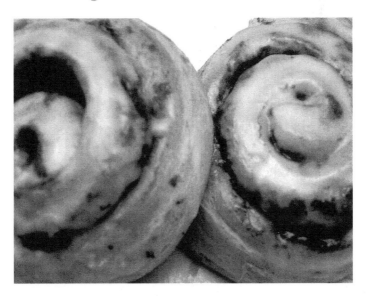

As doctors and researchers have looked for the best ways to use a low carb diet, they have expanded the information available.

A major advance for diabetic diet planning is the development of the glycemic index and the related concept of glycemic load.

The Glycemic Index (GI) is a rating system for foods where a food containing carbohydrate receives a numerical value based on its components and how each food affects the body's sugar levels. The GI value comes from tests on approximately 50 grams of a food.

The Glycemic Index uses pure glucose (or in some cases, white bread) as its control food and rates all other carbohydrates in relation to it. The control food or standard, either the glucose or the white bread, is given a rating of "100" and all other foods are tested as to how they affect a person's blood sugar, insulin and lipid levels compared to the standard.

Each tested food is given a number rating and defined as either "High", "Medium" or "Low" on the Glycemic Index. Foods fall into the High Glycemic Index when they are rated at 70 or above. If the Glycemic Index for a food is at 55 or lower, it is considered to be a Low Glycemic Index food item. This means that Medium Glycemic Index foods are those that after being tested, fall into the range of 56 to 69.

Foods such as unsweetened low fat yogurt, blackberries, peaches, almonds, and peanuts all score below 30, making them better choices when following a Glycemic Index diet. This means that they will not spike your blood sugar levels and may release energy slowly, over a longer period of time. This type of food will give you more energy, keep you feeling satisfied longer, and cut down the urge to binge on snack foods that are bad for your diabetes and for you.

Many of the lower glycemic index foods are also more likely to help you lower your total cholesterol or even change the balance of "bad" cholesterol (LDL) to "good" cholesterol (HDL) in your favor.

The Glycemic Load computes the amount of carbohydrate in the serving size portion of a given food eaten, versus the Glycemic Index value for 50 grams of the same food. You can calculate the Glycemic Load from a serving of food by multiplying the food's Glycemic Index rating with the number of grams of carbohydrates it contains in the serving size you are eating.

If the food's Glycemic Index Rating is below 100, use a decimal point to show that it is less than one. For instance, a baked potato has a high Glycemic Index rating of 85. The number of grams of carbohydrates in a medium baked potato is 37. By multiplying 0.85 and 37, we get just over 31. Therefore, a baked potato has a Glycemic Load of 31, making it a better choice in our diet than you might otherwise have thought.

The average range in the Glycemic Load is lower than the Glycemic Index. A food may be considered pretty high on the Glycemic Load ranking if it is above 50. The best recommendation is to keep the total number of your daily Glycemic Load to fewer than 150. This is much easier than counting calories or fat grams and it ensures that you are making the better choices for yourself in your diabetes self-care program.

As a practical matter, if a food is high in fat or fiber, those constituents will slow down the absorption of any carbohydrates in the serving consumed. Many diabetes educators advise patients on insulin to look at the total carbohydrates in a food, but then substract the grams of fat and fiber before calculating how much insulin to take. Otherwise, it is possible to take too much insulin for the net carbs that a given food can deliver into your system.

The GI charts below are not complete, but they give you a good idea about where many commonly-eaten foods stand.

Here are some charts, broken down by high, medium, and low GI ratings for each food.

HIGH GI – Avoid these foods

HIGH GLYCEMIC INDEX FOODS (OVER 70)	
FOOD	INDEX RATING
Bagel	72
Baked Potato	85
Cheerios	74
Cream of Wheat	74
Doughnut	76
French Fries	76
GatorAde	78
Graham Cracker	74
Honey	73
Jelly Beans	80
Mashed Potatoes	73
Rice Cakes	82
Rice Crispies	82
Rye Bread	76
Vanilla Wafers	77
Watermelon	72
White Bread	70

MEDIUM GI – Use these foods sparingly

MEDIUM GLYCEMIC INDEX FOODS (56-69)	
FOOD	INDEX RATING
Angel Food Cake	67
Beets	64
Blueberry Muffin	59
Bran Muffin	60
Cheese Pizza	60
Couscous	65
Hamburger Bun	61
Ice Cream	61
Mac & Cheese	64
Mini Shredded Wheat	58
Oatmeal	65
Orange Juice	56
Pea Soup	66
Peaches, canned	58
Pineapple	66
Pita Bread	57
Raisins	64
Rye Bread	68
Sourdough Bread	57
Taco Shells	69
Wheat Thins	67
White rice	56
Whole Wheat Bread	69

LOW GI – Choose these foods most often

LOW GLYCEMIC INDEX FOODS (UNDER 55)	
FOOD	INDEX RATING
Brown Rice	55
Apple Juice	41
Baked Beans	48
Banana	53
Broccoli	6
Carrots, cooked	39
Cauliflower	6
Cheese tortellini	50
Cherries, fresh	22
Chocolate	49
Fruit cocktail, canned	55
Grapefruit	25
Grapes	43
Ice Cream, low fat	50
Kidney Beans	52
Kiwifruit	52
Lentils	28
Lettuce	7
Linguine	55
Lowfat Yogurt, sweetened	33
Macaroni	45
Milk, fat free	32
Milk, Soy	30
Oatmeal Cookies	55
Oatmeal, old fashioned	49
Orange Juice, fresh	52
Peach, fresh	28
Peanuts	14
Peas	48
Popcorn	55
Potato Chips	54
Pound Cake	54
Snickers Bar	40
Spaghetti	41
Special K Cereal	54
Spinach	12
Sweet Corn	55
Sweet Potato	54
Tomato	15

Glycemic Index Recipe Sampler

Taking the matter beyond low carb eating to GI-based eating – check out the sample Glycemic Index recipes below. With food that tastes this good, you won't even realize it's healthy for you! Test out these glycemic index recipes today!

Chicken with Fried Rice

Ingredients:

12 fl. oz of chicken stock

1½ oz brown rice

5 ½ oz cooked chickpeas

2 fl. oz light soy sauce

1 tsp sesame oil

2 cubed boneless skinless chicken breasts

8 oz sliced mushrooms

1 green onion, chopped

1 carrot, diced

2 sticks sliced celery

8 oz bean sprouts

Salt, to taste (use herb seasoning if you prefer to limit your salt intake)

In a medium saucepan, add 10 fl. oz of your chicken stock, salt, and your rice. After it boils, reduce the heat to low and cook, covered, for about 25 minutes or until all of the liquid in the pot has been absorbed.

Fluff the rice with a fork, and set it aside.

In a large non-stick skillet, add sesame oil and heat over a medium to high eat. Cook the chicken the mushrooms for 8-10 minutes, or until the chicken is white all the way through.

Add the onions, celery, carrots, chickpeas, and rice. Stir thoroughly while cooking for about two minutes.

Add the rest of the chicken stock, along with the soy sauce, for another 5 minutes. Add the sprouts and mix.

Enjoy this delicious glycemic index recipe with a light salad!

Chicken Tarragon Delight

Ingredients:

2 chicken cutlets (Roughly 4 oz each)

2 teaspoons of vegetable oil

8 oz sliced mushrooms

2 oz. white wine

1 teaspoon of margarine

1 tsp. dried tarragon

Fresh ground pepper

1 small onion chopped

4 oz. chicken stock or water

In a non-stick pan, add oil and heat over a medium to high heat. Take the chicken and sprinkle with fresh ground pepper - then sauté in the oil until it's done. Remove the chicken and cover.

In that same pan, add the margarine and sauté both the mushrooms and the onions until they're soft, or for about five minutes. Then, add the wine and tarragon.

Let this mixture simmer for roughly a minute, then add the stock. Let it simmer for about two minutes, or until it's reduced itself to half. Add a bit of pepper to the mixture, and it's done!

Serve the sauce over chicken.

Suggestions: Looking for a great side with this? Serve this low GI recipe over brown rice (whose glycemic index is around 55 – and it brings in fiber and B vitamins as good nutrition too)!

Low Glycemic Index Chocolate Cookies

Ingredients:

3oz non-hydrogenated soft margarine

3oz wholegrain flour (look at low GI kamut also)

1 tablespoon of wheat or oat bran

Sugar substitute equivalent to about 4oz of sugar

¼ pint cooked white kidney beans

1½oz unsweetened cocoa powder

3 fl oz skim milk

1 egg

2 teaspoons of vanilla

½ teaspoon of baking soda

Add the beans, 1 fl. oz of skim milk, and wheat bran in a food processor. Puree until well blended.

Add the egg, vanilla, skim milk, baking soda, cocoa powder, sugar substitute, flour, margarine, and bean puree until a bowl, and beat it together until well mixed.

Preheat over to about 375 degrees. Drop the cookie batter from heaping teaspoons onto a wax paper-lined baking sheet. Bake them for about 10 minutes, or until they're firm.

Note: Not sure about the bean paste? You can't taste it, but it keeps the batter from drying out, and adds a little extra fiber into your diet!

For more glycemic index recipes, you can easily convert your favorite recipes to increase the fiber and protein content!

As you might have already guessed, the cinnamon buns in the beginning of this chapter are high in calories, carbs, and often fats. You may be able to make a low glycemic index, low glycemic load version of these – but steer clear of the commercial cinnamon buns. Just too much for a diabetic body to handle.

In contrast, the raspberries at the end of this chapter are a low glycemic fruit that brings in lots of beneficial nutrients, including antioxidants to protect your cells against the damaging effects of high blood sugars and diabetes. And, small portions of semi-sweet dark chocolate, with its high antioxidant levels and fat content to slow the sugar absorption, can be a delightful treat in moderation as well.

Your Action Steps:

1. Make a list of 3 low carb, low glycemic index foods that you will use to replace a higher carb food in your diet during the next week.

2. Find recipes for a week of low carb, low glycemic index (GI) eating, both meals and snacks.

3. If you don't already have one, buy a food scale and measuring cups to be able to measure the portions that you are eating, meal by meal.

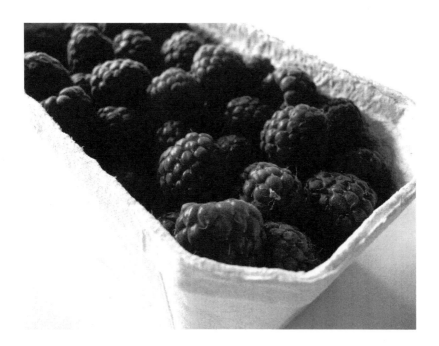

Superfoods for Better Blood Sugar Control

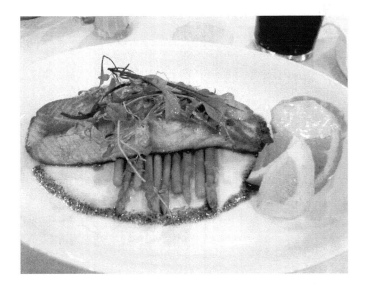

Superfoods are foods that have many health-promoting nutrients and very few downsides. In this chapter, we'll talk about good choices that are lower on the glycemic index (GI) rating scale and good for you.

Berries for Better Health

Berries include blueberries, cranberries, raspberries, and blackberries, among others. Each has some unique flavor, but all are low GI and tasty. Let's take blueberries as a good example.

Blueberries are one of the super foods we hear a lot about, and with good reason. These delicious, deep blue summer berries are well-known for their antioxidants, containing the highest amount of any other berries. However, blueberries have some other specific health benefits that are worth talking about. Let's take a look.

Health Benefits

The list of health benefits from eating blueberries is stacking up, and there aren't many parts of your body that couldn't benefit from a little extra blueberry goodness.

If you're looking for a low-calorie, high-fiber fruit with lots to offer your health, blueberries may be just what you need. One cup of blueberries has less than 100 calories, and offers one-quarter of your daily requirement for Vitamin C.

Loaded with vitamins and minerals, blueberries provide nutrients that are significant in keeping your brain healthy. Specifically, scientists claim that blueberries maintain and restore a healthy nervous system, prevent the death of brain cells that lead to health concerns like Alzheimer's disease, and keep your memory sharp for a long time. That's a lot of brain power.

Better vision is another benefit associated with consumption of blueberries, due to the fact that they contain compounds called anthocyanosides and flavonoids, which can slow down visual loss, as well as help prevent macular degeneration, myopia, and cataracts. Blueberries also have some heavy molecules which can help prevent urinary tract infections by washing away harmful bacteria.

Other important antioxidants are anthocyanins, known to benefit the prevention of heart and cardiovascular disease. Blueberries have been found to contain even more anthocyanins than red wine, long thought to be one of the better sources of this defender against free radicals. Even hemorrhoids, varicose veins, and peptic ulcers can benefit from the antioxidants found in these super berries.

A couple interesting cautions regarding blueberries are coming to light. Apparently, the protein in milk depletes the antioxidant power of the acids contained in blueberries. One study suggests that it is best to eat blueberries either one hour before or two hours after drinking milk. So, blueberries on your morning cereal may not be, nutritionally speaking, the wise thing to do. Instead, choose blueberries as a high-energy late morning snack or to top off a green salad.

Another interesting aspect of blueberries is that they contain oxalates, which can become concentrated and crystallize, creating some concern for those with a tendency for gallstones or kidney stones. Drinking enough water daily may help reduce the risk of kidney stones, though it may not prevent them.

As with other life choices, do all things in moderation and pay attention to allergies and other health concerns before indulging. But, for the vast majority, blueberries offer a wealth of nutrients that will benefit our health and well-being.

Choosing Blueberries

With so many health benefits, the question is not whether to eat blueberries, but how to eat them. First, you need to pick good specimens. Choose blueberries that are firm and uniform in color, not dull-looking or watery. Avoid packages that show white mold growth in the container – this can be an issue.

In fact, water will cause the berries to spoil more quickly, so they should be kept in dry containers in the refrigerator. For this reason, you'll also want to dry blueberries thoroughly after you wash them.

If you can't buy fresh, buy frozen. Blueberries freeze nicely and can be purchased whole or smashed. When you want to eat them, just thaw and enjoy. If frozen blueberries are used in cooking, you can thaw them or throw them into the recipe frozen and just adjust your cooking time slightly.

You'll find blueberry recipes in every section of a cookbook. From breakfast to breads, salads to sauces, and desserts to smoothie drinks, blueberries can be enjoyed from morning to night. Even without a cookbook handy, you can eat blueberries very simply as a 'one ingredient' super-food snack that is naturally sweet, but low GI.

If you're looking for an easy to eat super-food that is loaded with not only nutrition, but flavor and versatility, get to know this beautiful berry. Perfect as a snack, a dessert, or any number of dishes, blueberries definitely earn their place in your kitchen, and your healthy diet.

Broccoli: Disease-Fighting Vegetable

Today, broccoli remains one of the best selling vegetables in America for many reasons. This low-calorie, nutrient-rich vegetable gets respect for some miraculous health benefits. This list of benefits includes fighting cancer, boosting our immune systems, building stronger bones, and lowering the risk for cataracts. Broccoli earns its distinction as one of the top super foods in diets around the world.

Broccoli is a very good source of dietary fiber, vitamin A, vitamin C, vitamin K, B6, folate, potassium and manganese. We're familiar with most of these, of course, but did you know that folate is linked to reducing birth defects and heart disease? Along with these nutrients, broccoli is also a good source of protein, vitamin E, thiamin, riboflavin, calcium, and iron.

The words super-food and antioxidant often go together, and broccoli is no exception. Rich in antioxidants, those damaging free-radicals don't stand a chance against broccoli. One of those antioxidants is coenzyme Q10 which helps the body produce energy. Another specific component of broccoli's superfood status involves a compound called sulforaphane which triggers potent anti-cancer enzymes and may help protect against diabetes. These enzymes are also effective in eliminating bacteria that can cause peptic ulcers.

And, you don't have to eat a lot of broccoli to get all these super nutrients. Just one cup of broccoli provides over 40 milligrams of calcium and almost 80 milligrams of vitamin C. That even beats milk as a nutritional food source. All this nutrition is available in only 25 calories, and broccoli is very low in saturated fat and cholesterol.

Choosing the Right Bunch

Selecting fresh broccoli isn't difficult. Look for sturdy stalks with compact, dark green florets, and avoid wilted specimens with yellowing buds, as these stalks are already past their prime. Broccoli stores well in the refrigerator for up to three days before losing its vitamin content. In some supermarkets, you will even find hybrids like broccoflower or broccolini, which combine kale or cauliflower with broccoli.

Trim any leaves from the stalk and trim the woody end of the stalk off the bottom. If you prefer to eat only the florets, or your recipe calls for just the florets, cut the broccoli florets off the stalk, rinse under running water, and drain. Save the stalks for another recipe if desired.

Broccoli Cooking and Serving Ideas

Broccoli is one of the more versatile vegetables you can eat, holding up well in a number of recipes and cooking methods. Of course, the closer you keep your broccoli to its raw state, the more nutrients you will maintain.

If you are cooking your broccoli to serve as a side dish, you should only cook it for a few moments, until the florets turn bright green. Cooking broccoli for more time than necessary causes the nutritional benefits to deteriorate. If the broccoli becomes mushy during steaming or boiling, it has cooked too long.

You may choose to flash-cook the broccoli in a microwave to keep the cooking time short and to maintain more of the nutrients. Of course, the microwave debate still goes on about whether it reduces or destroys nutrients in broccoli. You decide. If using the microwave is the only way you'll get around to making broccoli, then use it.

Broccoli can be used in anything from stir-fry to casseroles, omelets, soups, and salads. The florets are a pretty and nutritious addition to many dishes.

The stalks can be chopped and sauted, roasted, or cooked and pureed for a creamy broccoli soup. Use the broccoli florets to eat a low carb bean dip. You'll find thousand of recipes using broccoli once you start searching.

Of course, we can't talk about broccoli and kids without talking about broccoli trees. Raw broccoli florets look like little trees, so use this to your advantage when trying to get kids to eat their broccoli. With a bit of creamy dressing for 'snow,' make a little forest of broccoli trees and your kids will be tempted to gobble them up in no time. For adults eating low carb meals, use a low carb dressing.

It should also be noted that sprouts from broccoli have the same healthful benefits as the plant itself. Toss a handful of sprouts on top of a salad for a real boost of flavor and nutrients. Or, tuck a pile of broccoli sprouts into a tortilla wrap sandwich for a crunchy treat. Anywhere you want to add crunch, add broccoli sprouts.

No matter how you serve broccoli - raw, blanched, or steamed as a side dish, or as an ingredient in a main dish, you can't go wrong with this powerhouse vegetable.

Besides the boost broccoli gives your immune system, and your overall health, broccoli is just plain tasty. This is one super food you don't want to skip.

Beans: Vegetable Protein with High Fiber

Beans (legumes) are an excellent food to give you fiber, protein, and necessary nutrients such as B vitamins (B1, B2, and niacin). Different beans have different types of advantages. Pinto beans, for instance, also have calcium, phosphorus, potassium and iron.

Recent studies have shown that people who eat a high vegetable protein diet do better in terms of heart disease and other health outcomes than those who focus on a high protein animal protein diet. Beans also are a less costly way to nourish your body.

There aren't a lot of foods that can hold more than one place on the food pyramid. But, long before we started talking about "super foods," ancient peoples knew the benefits this humble food had to offer -- as a vegetable, a protein, and a healer.

In traditional Indian medicine, there exists an age-old system of living and healing that includes a vegetarian diet using legumes like lentils, beans, and peas to keep the body healthy.

Now, beyond other cultures, many people recognize the power of the bean to support whole nutrition and well-being. Here, we discuss some of the benefits of beans, and why they are leading a double life as a well respected super food.

Perfect Nutrition on Many Levels

Legumes are edible seeds contained in pods, and beans are part of that family. By their very nature, beans have a convenience factor that makes them a favorite food in many parts of the world. They are generally inexpensive and store well with the potential for a long shelf life, particularly when they are dried. Beans offer sustained nutrition and energy due to the fact they have a low glycemic index, meaning they provide energy to the body over a long period of time.

You won't get bored quickly eating beans, either. There is virtually an endless variety of beans and legumes to choose from, as well as a mountain of recipes to try when adding beans to your healthy diet. A short list of beans would include navy beans, black beans, lentils, soybeans, great northern beans, mung beans, garbanzo beans, pinto beans, black eyed peas, and kidney beans.

Beans are an excellent source of dietary fiber, minerals, and vitamins, and are naturally low in fat, calories, and sodium. You can serve beans in nutritious main dishes or side dishes that will satisfy your appetite with less-costly consequences to your body, or budget. These reasons alone would easily earn beans their super food status, but there's more!

Eating several servings of beans each day not only helps you reach your daily vegetable requirement, but those same beans also add up as your protein intake. Yes, those inexpensive, versatile beans are a protein. That's why we consider them a double-duty super food. Beans can easily be combined in recipes with other protein sources, vegetables, and starches like corn, whole wheat, or brown rice to create 'complete proteins' containing all the necessary amino acids our bodies require to function well.

Good Health Contributions

Beans have numerous healthy qualities that make them excellent additions to any diet. As we mentioned, not only are beans a nutritious vegetable source, but a perfect choice as a meat substitute. By reducing high-fat protein sources like red meats in your diet, and substituting low fat beans as your source of protein, you are fighting high cholesterol, high blood pressure, as well as a host of other ailments that can occur from a diet high in fat.

Antioxidants battle those nasty free radicals, the cell damaging agents in your body, and beans have some of the highest antioxidant content of any food on the planet. Although the benefits vary between different types of beans, all beans help regulate blood pressure and blood sugar levels, lower cholesterol, and improve digestion. The dietary fiber and enzymes in beans have the added benefit of helping to block cancer-causing cells and compounds in the intestines and colon.

The humble little kidney bean contains a healthy dose of thiamin, which regulates memory and brain function. Many beans also contain isoflavones, which can ease menopause symptoms and improve bone and prostate health, just to name a few benefits. Choose any bean and you've chosen a super food well worth the title.

Unlimited Possibilities

Beans can be cooked in countless dishes like chili, stew, soup, stir fry, tacos, salads, casseroles, and omelets. Try your hand at several main dishes or side dishes and explore your options. Don't limit yourself to just the classic beans and rice dish. Choose a new salad or a tasty dip for chips. Hot, cold, mashed, or whole, the bean will constantly surprise you with its versatility.

As opposed to canned beans, dried beans are the cheapest way to have this super food on hand. In general, cooking dried beans is easy. Rinse your dried beans, cover in water and soak overnight. Then, set the beans in a big pot, cover them with fresh water, bring to a boil and simmer for about an hour or so until they are soft. You can skip soaking them overnight, just increase the cooking time to about two hours. You will also find many recipes for cooking dried beans in a crockpot or pressure cooker. Do a bit of research or follow the directions on the package of beans for best results.

Soaking beans well will also help soften the fiber and reduce the gas that some people experience when they first start on a higher bean containing det. If that does not help enough, there are many products on the market to help digest the fiber that can cause the gas during digestion.

No matter how you choose to eat this super food, your body will thank you. You can eat enough beans to satisfy even the heartiest appetite without worrying about fat or calories. Beans are economical, a great source of dietary fiber, and are loaded with vitamins and minerals.

Besides all that good news, a bag of beans in your pantry means you've always got protein with a long shelf life in your house, too. As far as super foods go, beans easily make it to the top of the list.

Omega-3 Fatty Acid Foods: Fish and Flax

First, let's try to understand a bit of brain science. The brain is made up of about sixty percent fat. This fat is found mainly within the membranes that surround the brain's nerve cells. The composition and chemistry of these membranes has a direct effect on chemical reactions in the brain.

These chemical reactions are the brain's signals. The influence that more Omega 3 in the fat has on these signals has been studied extensively. It is believed that Omega 3 fatty acids promote better and faster transfer of signals in the brain. Okay. I guess that means Omega 3 fatty acids are good for you. Let's see how.

When your brain signals are working well, your whole body benefits. Besides brain health itself, other health benefits related to Omega 3s include inhibiting cancer cell growth, reducing inflammation throughout the body, prohibiting excess clotting in the blood, and reducing the risk of obesity by stimulating a hormone called leptin, which helps regulate metabolism and body weight.

As a diabetic, you want to be especially focused on choosing foods that cut down chronic inflammation, reduce clotting risk, and help you lose weight.

While there is some debate over the true ability of Omega 3s in treating or improving things like mental disorders, heart disease, and cancer, many researchers still claim there are significant benefits to consuming foods that contain these vital fats.

Where to Find Sources of Omega-3 Fatty Acids

If you live in Alaska, Taiwan, or Japan you may already be eating enough foods rich in Omega 3 fatty acids. The reason is that these populations routinely consume fish that is fatty, in a good way. Diets that contain fatty fish are continuing to show better results with respect to less inflammatory ailments and less obesity-related diseases, such as diabetes and heart disease.

But, if you don't live in one of those areas, you can still find plenty of the Omega 3s you need. These fatty acids are most prevalent in seafoods, with wild salmon, tuna, scallops, sardines, and trout being particularly rich. Other sources of Omega 3s are algae, krill, shrimp, and tofu, as well as certain nuts and seeds, like walnuts and flaxseeds.

Other vegetables and spices like cloves, mustard seeds, cauliflower, collard greens, and cabbage are good sources for Omega 3s. Even certain berries, like strawberries and raspberries, provide at least some of the same healthy benefits.

Let's take salmon as a good example of a high protein source of omega-3s. The mighty salmon is probably one of the most widely studied fish we know. These studies often involve sustainability and contaminants comparing farmed salmon with wild caught salmon.

Farmed salmon represents a large majority of available fish in the U.S. However, these farmed salmon have been treated with antibiotics, have more fat content, and have less beneficial omega 3. For these reasons alone, wild salmon is a much healthier choice for regular consumption.

Salmon is categorized as a 'fatty' fish, but don't let that scare or confuse you. The fat that is referred to is where we find the most powerful super food imaginable – omega 3 fatty acids (the good fats). These fatty acids are essential nutrient elements that contribute to your body's healthy functioning, beginning right at the top with the brain, and continuing throughout the body.

And, you can get more omega 3 fatty acids in just one 4 ounce serving of salmon than you would get in several days of trying to eat other healthy foods containing some omega 3s.

With so much emphasis on the tremendous amount and availability of omega 3 fatty acids in salmon, some of the other healthy aspects have tended to be overlooked. Salmon is rich in tryptophan, the amino acid that helps the nervous system relax, rest, and even sleep.

With more than 100 IU's of vitamin D in a serving of salmon, you have one of the very best sources available. Also, salmon is an excellent source of selenium, which is associated with decreased risk of joint inflammation, prevention of certain types of cancer, and is known to protect against cardiovascular diseases.

And that's not all. Don't forget the protein. Salmon, like other fish, is a great, good fat, low calorie source of protein. Then you get B3 (niacin), B12, B6, phosphorus, and magnesium. And not just minimal amounts either... you're getting serious doses of nutrients in this seriously delicious fish.

More Salmon Benefits

As you can see, salmon has a lot to offer, but along with all those vitamins, minerals, and omega 3s, salmon is also lower in cholesterol than other seafood and shellfish, like shrimp and lobster. So, while the omega 3s are improving cardiovascular health, the salmon is not adding a lot of cholesterol to counteract all the benefits.

The all-important omega 3s we've been talking about in salmon not only contribute to better brain function and memory, but also supports skin health, joint health, heart health, and digestive health, along with a host of other benefits. Experts recommend 1-2 meals of fish per week.

Salmon also has selenium and certain amino acids that protect the nervous system from the effects of the aging process. It is also known to lower the risk of Parkinson and Alzheimer's disease, and can help prevent blood clots that can contribute to stroke.

Salmon tends to speed up the metabolism, which helps regulate blood sugar levels in the body. That little four ounce serving of salmon we talked about earlier provides up to 30 grams of protein, which we know supports muscle strength. But, don't forget about one of our most important muscles – the heart. Yes, salmon has a lot of offer every system of our body. But, how can you enjoy salmon a couple times a week without getting tired of it?

Preparing Super Salmon Dishes

A broiled, baked, or grilled salmon fillet is delicious all on its own, for most fish lovers. But for some, the unique flavor of salmon is better when fixed in slightly different dishes or with a variety of sauces.

Cooked salmon works well with a lot of flavors. A number of different glazes and seasonings can turn each salmon experience into a unique one. Some herbs and spices to try in your rubs or sauces include cayenne pepper, mustard, fennel, ginger, and paprika.

A classic sauce for salmon that's worthy of your time is a maple syrup glaze (diabetics: look for no carb syrup such as Walden Farms' brand). Made simply by combining a mixture of Walden Farms low calorie/no carb maple syrup with various ingredients like stevia, lemon juice, Dijon mustard, and even chili powder, this sauce makes a splendidly sweet and savory glaze that compliments the salmon perfectly without undermining your health.

Creamed soups are another good option for enjoying salmon. Much like lobster bisque, salmon bisque has a rich flavor that can be slightly sweet, slightly spicy, and definitely delicious. Keep this bisque simple as the flavor of the salmon will carry it just fine.

Salmon that has been cooked, cooled, and tossed in a big salad with mixed greens is a great choice for folks who like a little crunch surrounding their salmon. Choose a light vinaigrette and a variety of vegetables for your salmon salads.

One vegetable that is especially complementary with salmon is cucumbers. Try making a simple flaked salmon and diced cucumber sandwich spread for something extra special. Just mix in a bit of light mayonnaise and spread on toasted low carb, whole grain (yes, you can find this type) English muffins or hearty whole grain crackers.

Of course, a favorite for holidays and buffet tables is smoked salmon. A few pieces of smoked salmon on a hearty multigrain cracker is enough to convince most non-believers that salmon is a food to favor. But, you can also used smoked salmon to create wonderful salads, spreads, and more. There is really no end to the ways you can enjoy this super super-food.

This popular fish lends itself to lots of different ideas and recipes, so don't be afraid to experiment with new flavors to find the ones you like best. Salmon is a super healthy food that provides countless beneficial nutrients all wrapped up in a super tasty fish.

Generally speaking, eating a healthy diet rich in green leafy vegetables, lean meats, seafood, as well as nuts and berries, contributes to better health. This general guide just happens to include many foods that are naturally rich in Omega 3 fatty acids. That could be one of the simplest ways to supplement your good health, and it's all right on your dinner plate!

Oats: Healthy Whole Grain Food

Oats gained a special distinction as a super food back in 1997 when the Food and Drug Administration made the claim that there is an association between a diet high in oats and a reduced risk of coronary heart disease.

With that announcement, oats, oatmeal, oat bran, and oat flour skyrocketed in popularity among the whole grains, placing it right up there in the top 10 super foods. Let's take a look at what else this well known, but not totally understood, grain has to offer.

Impressive Nutritional Value

We know that oats, along with other whole grains, provide protection against heart disease, potentially extending the lifespan of people who include this food regularly in their diets. That would seem to be enough of a reason to add whole grain oats to your diet, but there's more.

This is a high fiber, high protein, low glycemic index food that's low in calories and rich in important vitamins and minerals like iron, calcium, copper, potassium, manganese, and selenium.

Beta glucan is the main ingredient responsible for lowering serum cholesterol levels. Oats also contain special antioxidants called avenanthramides. Together these two elements have been shown to significantly reduce LDL cholesterol levels when oats are consumed on a regular basis. Lowering "bad" LDL cholesterol is a big plus for anyone with diabetes.

Oats have a low glycemic index which means the energy from this food burns slowly and stays with you to satisfy your hunger for a longer period of time. Having nutrients released slowly into the bloodstream and throughout the body helps stabilize blood sugar levels, eliminating the spikes which can cause many health problems, concentration problems, and dieting problems. In addition, the B vitamins contribute to strong healthy skin, nails, hair, and brain function.

Along with other whole grains, studies have found that consuming oats can aid in the battle against type 2 diabetes, breast cancer, and asthma in children. With this sort of super food on your side, why wouldn't you eat it?

Countless Recipes

Oats are an inexpensive and widely available grain that can be easily incorporated into meals at any time of day. Oats are easy to store in containers or airtight bags, and have a very long shelf life.

A bowl of hot cereal in the morning is the most familiar way oats are served. Whether you buy raw oatmeal or quick cooking, you are starting off with a good basis for nutrition. Vary the toppings and you vary the recipe enough to eat servings of oatmeal a number of times each week without getting bored. Add berries, nuts, stevia, or protein powders to boost the flavor and superpowers of your oatmeal.

Besides breakfast cereal, there are a number of other ways to incorporate oats into your daily diet. Oats can provide a toasty coating for baked or broiled fish, and are often used to make hearty muffins, cookies, and other desserts. Don't forget about convenient trail mixes or granola bars. Oats are often the central ingredient in those tasty treats.

Mixing oatmeal in as a binder in ground meat for burgers, meatloaf, and meatballs is another way to 'sneak' more nutrition into your diet. Oats also play center stage in a number of bread recipes, whether as a main ingredient or to add just a bit of heartiness and crunch.

As part of your healthy diet, incorporating up to three servings of whole grains a day is recommended by many nutritionists and health experts. Oats provide enough significant benefits for healthy living to make them a vital part of your good diet.

Nuts Are Remarkable Super Foods

Nuts like almonds, walnuts, pecans, and pistachio nuts have great health promoting benefits. That little nut you have been snacking on is really a super food because of the unique combination of fats, protein, vitamins, and minerals. This tiny powerhouse works hard lowering the risk of some major diseases and health conditions.

Don't let the fat content or calorie count of nuts worry you too much. Even though nuts are often high in calories and fat, they have 'good' fats and omega 3 fatty acids that lower "bad" cholesterol levels and help regulate blood pressure and healthy heart rhythms. The fiber content in nuts also helps control cholesterol and has been found to lower the risk for diabetes.

But that's not all. Certain types of nuts also have plant sterols which is another cholesterol inhibitor. So important as a cholesterol inhibitor, as a matter of fact, that plant sterols are added to things like orange juice and margarine for the health benefits. And you've got it all right there in a nut.

In addition, vitamin E and the amino acid L-arginine are two elements that help reduce plaque in the circulatory system, which helps to prevent clots in arteries. Nuts have so many of these healthy elements that they may be one of the most powerful foods you can eat to take care of your heart.

Enjoy Nuts in Numerous Ways

The important thing to remember with nuts is, like many other things in life, too much of a good thing isn't really good. Since nuts are dense in calories and fat, a little goes a long way. For instance, just a dozen or so cashews can have up to 180 calories.

For this reason, health experts recommend limiting your daily intake of most nuts to no more than a couple of ounces. This is actually good news for your budget, since adding nuts to your healthy diet requires only a small investment for such a big return.

So, what specific nuts are best to eat regularly? There isn't really a lot of definitive research to suggest one type of nut is better than another. Walnuts, almonds, pistachioos, pecans, peanuts (which are really in the legume family), and cashews are popular and easy to find in most regions. Cashews are a bit higher in carb content than other nuts, so limit that specific nut if possible.

You'll also find many recipes for these various nuts, so it's easy to incorporate nuts into your meals as well as your snacking.

Consider substituting chopped nuts for chocolate chips in cookies, for example. Toss peanuts into a green salad or pasta salad for added nutrition and crunch. Use natural peanut butter on your morning toast instead of butter or jam. Walnuts are a classic choice to top a savory salad. Chop almonds up and toss in your vanilla yogurt for a nice crunch. Grab a bag of pistachios to have a healthy snack in late afternoon at work.

You can also grind almonds, peanuts, or other nuts into a coarse meal. Use this meal to coat chicken or fish instead of using the higher GI cornmeal or white flour when frying or baking. Grind the meal fine and add to smoothies in your blender.

Almonds can be ground into a flour consistency and can be used in many dishes as a substitute for wheat flour. This gluten-free flour alternative has become very popular in recent years. You can also find unsweetened almond milk as a great milk substitute if you don't tolerate cow's milk or soy milk.

It's best to buy shelled, unsalted, or minimally processed varieties of nuts in small quantities. You can also protect fresh nuts from oxidation by storing them in a cool, dark, dry place. Or you can store nuts in an airtight container in the refrigerator or freezer. The oils that naturally occur in nuts can become rancid if exposed to heat and air.

Adding small amounts of nuts to your diet will provide your body with big benefits. Choose a variety of nuts, store them properly, and enjoy a handful of crunchy nutrition every day.

Just make sure that you are not allergic to the type of nuts you choose. Peanut allergy is the best known, and it can cause a very serious life-threatening reaction in susceptible people. But, if you tolerate nuts, include them in your low carb diet. These are truly a super food.

Your Action Steps:

1. Choose at least 3 superfoods from the list in this chapter that you have not eaten in the past month.

2. Design your weekly menu plan to include each of the foods you have chosen.

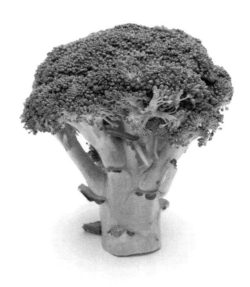

Low Carb Recipe Sampler

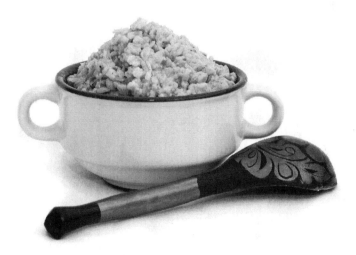

Low carb recipes do not necessarily use all low GI foods, but they give you a good start on easing yourself into a better way to plan your diabetic diet.

Low Carb Breakfast – Hearty Oatmeal

Oatmeal (regular – not instant oatmeal) in the morning is a good low carb, high fiber breakfast alternative if you want a hot breakfast, but not eggs. Whole grain oats can help lower high cholesterol too.

This can easily be made in the microwave.

Ingredients:

110g (1/2 c for one serving) whole grain original oatmeal
450ml water (1 c for one serving)
225ml (1/2 c for one serving) skimmed milk or soya milk or almond milk (unsweetened vanilla flavor)
Sprinkle cinnamon to taste (it will help control your blood sugar – and it tastes great too!)
1-2 drops of liquid Stevia sweetener or 2g artificial sweetener (optional)

Combine the oatmeal and water in a microwave safe bowl and cook on high for 4 minutes. Stir in the milk and sweetener if used and divide between 2 bowls.

If preparing on the stove, combine the oatmeal and water in a saucepan and bring to the boil over a medium heat. Reduce the heat and cook for a further 5 minutes, stirring occasionally. Stir in the milk and sweetener, divide between 2 bowls.

For those who prefer a cold meal in the mornings, plain or flavored low carb yogurt is a good breakfast option. Combining the yogurt with a cup of nuts or frozen berries or flax seed makes a quick low carb breakfast option.

Low carb shakes are another quick option that will keep you satisfied for some time. These can be bought already prepared from health stores or you can make your own.

Blend together a cup of milk or soya milk or almond milk (unsweetened vanilla) with 1 scoop of vanilla or chocolate low carb protein powder (use rice protein if milk casein allergic), half a cup of coconut milk, 2 tablespoons flax seed, sweetener to taste and 3-4 ice cubes.

Low Carb Lunch Ideas

Lunch time can often be a problem for many people. Whether you are at work or home, most of us tend to grab a snack at lunch time, usually in the form of an easy to make or buy sandwich.

However, if you are on a low carb diet, bread is usually not an option. Here, think about a selection of ideas for a low carb lunch that can just as easily be made to take to work or for a low carb lunch at home.

Salads are a popular choice for someone on a low carb diet. Salads need not be a boring plate of lettuce and cheese on a low carb diet. Use lots of salad greens such a arugula, spinach and watercress. Add crunch with nuts.

These not only add a lovely peppery flavor to a salad, but contain a good variety of nutrients than lettuce. Many salads can be bought pre-prepared. So when buying for a low carb lunch, having a bag in the fridge is very convenient.

You are only limited by your imagination as to what goes into your salad. Cold meats such as chicken, beef, pork make a filling low carb lunch.

Fish such as salmon and tuna (tinned or fresh) or seafood, not only make a filling high protein lunch, but provide you with essential vitamins, minerals, and omega-3 fatty acids. A Greek salad using feta cheese and extra eggs for protein or the classic Caesar salad are easy to prepare and pack for work.

If you need a choice of low carb, low calorie salad dressings, track down Walden Farms brand products in your local health food store or online. Many of these products will satisfy you need for taste and even texture – without affecting your blood sugar.

This same company also makes low carb, no calorie pancake syrups and chocolate dips and syrups. The availability of these kinds of foods gives you no excuse for eating high carb, high glycemic index foods that shoot your blood sugar sky high. You have good alternatives.

When on any diet it is important to have variety to stop boredom creeping in, so try to vary your low carb lunch menu. Adding flavor to your salads helps make them more interesting. So if using chicken in your salad, think about having chicken tikka or grilled chicken marinated in your favorite herbs and spices.

Adding a dressing to your salad is another way to add interest and flavor. If using bottled dressings always check the labels for carb values first by looking at the grams of carbohydrates. Many branded salad dressings have a high carb value. But there are many salad dressings you can make up yourself.

Using olive oil as a salad dressing is very versatile. Olive oil (which is anti-inflammatory health-promoting as an added benefit) can be bought with herbs such as basil and garlic already added. Keep a bottle at work to pour over your salad at the last moment to keep it crisp and fresh.

One very simple dressing that goes with many low carb lunch salads is lime dressing. You will need: 1 tablespoon lime juice, 1 teaspoon water, 2 tablespoons extra virgin olive oil, seasoning to taste and some sweetener to taste. Put the lime juice and water in a bowl and add the sweetener. Season to taste and whisk together. Whisk in the olive oil.

Olive oil is an especially health-promoting oil that reduces inflammation, unlike some other sources of fats. It is part of the well-known Mediterranean diet that research has shown can cut your risk of heart disease and other health conditions.

For those who prefer something hot for their low carb lunch, soup provides a complete meal in a bowl. There a very few ready made soups that are low carb, so, if buying soup, read the label first. Miso soup is one low carb soup. Low carb soup is a great way to use up leftovers. Make up a big batch and freeze it to have a ready supply of low carb lunches. There are many low carb soup recipes on line and in recipe books.

If cooking chicken, a delicious base for a soup is the chicken stock. Boil the bones from the chicken for at least half an hour, longer if you have time. Strain through a sieve and either cool and freeze for later or use straight away for your soup.

Frying some onions or leeks and adding low carb vegetables such as mushrooms and peppers and then blending them together with the chicken stock makes a very comforting low carb lunch.

Eggs are another great low carb lunch that are quick and easy to prepare. Omelettes can be loaded with many different low carb ingredients such as cheese, ham, mushrooms, peppers or low carb vegetables. Or have scrambled egg in a low carb tortilla topped with cheese.

Of course if you have to eat out at work it is not all that easy to find a low carb restaurant or snack bar. But with a little thought you can choose somewhere to eat that has low carb foods on the menu.

For instance, at a steak restaurant, you could have the steak and a green salad or grilled chicken or salmon. Many pizza places have very good salads -- just make sure you ask for the dressing on the side. And yes, you can have a burger -- just don't eat the bun. Some fast food places will make you a "protein style" burger wrapped in lettuce – juicy, tasty, and low carb.

For those wishing to buy a low carb lunch or low carb fast food ready prepared there are many low carb protein shakes and low carb bars on the market.

Low carb protein bars provide a quick snack. While this is not sufficient for a daily meal, they are handy to have in an emergency and can be kept in the office drawer or kitchen cupboard.

One of the best ways to make sure you have a low carb lunch ready is by using leftovers. When you make a main meal think about making a little extra or saving some for your lunch. Simply put it in a plastic container in the fridge for the next day or freeze batches for another time. This way you can build up a varied selection of 'ready meals'.

There are many low carb recipes on line to help you choose your low carb lunch. Being prepared for your week ahead also helps you stick to your low carb diet. Make a menu plan for the week and shop for the ingredients you will need. This is also a good way to save waste.

Low Carb Hearty Tomato Soup (gluten-free, dairy-free)

Ingredients:

1 can diced tomatoes (no added sugar), run through blender to leave chunks
1 8-ounce can tomato sauce (no added sugar)
Season with crushed garlic clove or garlic powder to taste, basil flakes, and/or oregano (if you want an Italian seasoning type of flavor)

Prepare by mixing all ingredients together in a pan and heat.

If you must have sweetener, add a drop of Stevia to the finished product, but this is optional

This is a quick, easy recipe for homemade soup. Make it in quantity and take it as part of your low carb lunches to reheat in a microwave.

Low Carb Bread (Gluten-Free)

Ingredients:

2 ½ cups of almond flour (blanched almond type)
½ teaspoon baking soda
½ tsp. salt (sea salt is best)
3 eggs
1 tablespoon agave nectar or Lo Han Sweetener (healthier with low glycemic index – but amount depends on which company's product you get – check label)
½ tsp. apple cider vinegar

Combine dry ingredients together in one bowl.
In a separate bowl, prepare the eggs with a whisk before adding the agave and vinegar.

Add wet ingredients into the drug ingredients and stir while adding.

Grease a loaf pan (should fit a 6 by 3 inch pain).
Put the batter into the greased pan.

Heat oven to 300 degrees.

Bake on low oven rack for 45-55 minutes. Test to make sure cake tester or knife comes out clean.
Cool before slicing or serving.

Low Carb New York Ricotta Cheesecake Dessert

This cheesecake is not for everyday desserts, with its calorie and fat counts, but this dessert can be a lower carb treat on special occasions.

Ingredients:

24 ounces cream cheese, softened
1 cup extra fine whole milk ricotta cheese. *This can be refined using a food processor for 1 minute.*
1/2 cup sour cream
1 1/2 cups splenda or equivalent stevia
1/3 cup heavy or double cream
1 Tbsp no sugar added vanilla extract
1 Tbsp fresh lemon juice
2 eggs
3 egg yolks
1 8-inch springform cake tin

Preheat oven to 400F

First you need to prepare your springform tin.Spray the tin with non-stick cooking spray and set aside. Using a shallow roasting tin big enough to hold the tin, fill about 1 inch of water and place the tray on the center shelf of the oven to pre-heat.

In a bowl beat together the cream cheese, ricotta, sour cream, and sweetener for about one minute using an electric mixer.

In a separate bowl, using a wire whisk mix the heavy cream, vanilla, lemon juice, eggs and egg yolks until well blended.

Turn the mixer onto a medium speed and slowly pour the egg mixture into the cream cheese mixture. Mix until just blended, being careful not to over-whip.

Pour the mixture into the springform tin and place into the heated roasting tin water bath.

Bake for 15 minutes and then lower the oven temperature to 275F and bake for 1 1/2 hours. The top should be a light golden brown and the cake should be pulling away from the sides.

Turn the oven off and leave the cake to cool in the oven for about 3 hours. Then remove the cake and refrigerate before serving.

12 servings

Sugarless Cake

Ingredients:

1 c. dates, chopped
1 c. prunes, chopped
1 c. raisins
1 c. cold water
1 stick margarine, melted
2 eggs
1 tsp. baking soda
1/4 tsp. salt
1 c. plain flour or flour substitute (almond, soy, pea, etc)
1 c. nuts, chopped
1/4 tsp. cinnamon
1/4 tsp. nutmeg
1 tsp. vanilla

Boil dates and prunes in the one cup of water for 3 minutes; add margarine and raisins and let cool.

Mix flour, soda, salt, eggs, nuts, spices and vanilla. Add to fruit mixture. Stir to blend.

Pour into baking dish. Bake at 350 degrees for 25 to 30 minutes.

More Low Carb & Good Carb Recipe Resources

Find More Recipes at:
www.HighBloodSugarSolution.com/get-more-recipes

Herbs for Diabetes

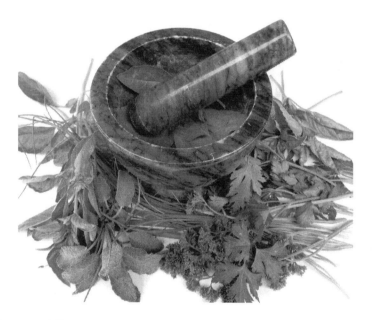

Green Tea

For those who are looking for new ways to control their blood sugar and potential damaging effects of diabetes, green tea is a simple way to support good health. Studies have shown that drinking green tea might be a way to not only regulate sugar, but also to prevent problems like cataracts, which are more likely in diabetic patients. Green tea offers help with preventing problems for those with diabetes.

Switching to Green Tea

The chemical makeup of green tea allows your body to more easily manage your blood sugar levels. When you drink green tea, you will be able to sustain a normal range of blood sugar, while helping to keep the levels steady. If you're a coffee drinker, it might be a good idea to start switching out your daily cup for green tea, eventually replacing your coffee habit altogether. Even if you're not willing to switch completely over to green tea, it's a good idea to add a few cups of tea a day to support your diabetes and weight control.

Other Benefits of Drinking Green Tea

In addition to helping prevent cataracts, green tea can help diabetics in other ways:

Support weight loss – Since being overweight can increase your risk of diabetic troubles, or even cause Type 2 diabetes in some patients, losing weight can be helpful. With green tea, you can reduce your appetite, while also increasing fat loss, according to some case studies.

Lower blood sugar – Those who have Type 2 diabetes find that drinking green tea can help to decrease the chances of blood sugar spikes, which can cause damage to the body.

Diabetes prevention – While studies are still being done on green tea, some initial findings indicate that green tea may prevent or slow the progression of Type 2 diabetes.

Improved concentration – If you find that your diabetes has caused you to have troubles with your memory or focus, green tea can also help support you.

In order to get the most effects from green tea, it's ideal that you drink this on a regular basis, avoiding adding sweeteners or milk to the brew. If you're concerned about the added caffeine consumption, you should note that green tea actually has less caffeine than coffee or black tea. It is also possible to get decaf green tea if you are very sensitive to the effects of caffeine.

Some experts have pointed out that drinking black tea can also be helpful for those with diabetes, but green tea seems to offer something that other teas cannot- ECCG.

This ingredient works with the body to help with blood sugar, and can even be helpful for those who are starting to show signs of pre-diabetes. Simple, cheap, and effective, adding green tea to your diet will allow you the chance to change your health today.

Bitter Melon (Foo Gwa)

Bitter melon is a plant that has shown promise because it actually blocks or prevents sugar absorption from occurring in the intestinal tract. Researchers in Asia have explored prolonged use of bitter melon as a form of diabetic control and discovered that a 90 day testing period of the compound did result in a lowering of glucose levels in most of the study group. This is a compound often found in the form of a "juice" and which is taken in doses of no more than 100 milliliters daily.

Bitter melon is a type of tropical vegetable from Asia, East Africa, and South America that is part of many home remedies or folk remedies for diabetes. At least the Asian form of bitter melon in research studies has shown that it can lower blood glucose levels, perhaps from the actions of several different compounds found naturally in the vegetable.

Make sure to ask your doctor before trying any herb, as many can interact with drugs you are taking and change the blood levels of the drugs up or down or cause other types of side effects such as diarrhea.

This herb comes straight from the traditions of Chinese medicine. It may lower insulin resistance. Research scientists isolated 4 specific bioactive components, which apparently activate AMPK, a protein in enzyme form that facilitates glucose uptake and stabilizes fuel metabolism.

Bitter Melon looks like a striking green, knobby squash, with a stringy, pithy center. It was used as early as the 16th century by famous Chinese physician Li Shizhen.

If you do manage to find some in your area, do check with your doctor first, of course. It is available in capsule form. Sometimes in traditional Chinese weddings, it may even be used as a vegetable in a pork dish.

Gymnema Syvestre

Gymnema Syvestre is a plant referred to as a sugar "destroyer" because it has demonstrated such proficiency for stimulating the natural enzymes that use up glucose. This means that you are reducing your need to rely on insulin to regulate blood sugar -- and this means that the risks of diabetic problems go down. This herb is found in a tablet form and is recommended at a 20 milligram dosage per day.

Gymnema Syvestre is from the tropical forests in India and is an ancient folk remedy for diabetes. Apparently this herb can lower blood sugar in both type 1 and type 2 diabetics.

Remember that while you want things that can help lower blood sugar, their effects could cause your usual doses of medication to become excessive — and you could end up with too low a blood sugar unless and until your doctor adjusts your medication doses.

That is why is it is very important to let your doctor know what you are doing and ask for help making these adjustment in drugs. Don't make changes on your own — many conventional drugs leave you with severe rebounds if you try to stop them too quickly.

There are several combination herbal products you can find with this key herbal ingredient, along with other herbs to protect other body parts from high blood sugar.

Prickly Pear (Opuntia)

Though this can be found as a food source in many grocery stores, Prickly Pear is best used as a supplement. In a range of studies, this herbal/plant compound has been shown to reduce blood sugar levels due to its natural contents that operate in much the same way as insulin.

Long used by Hispanic Americans in conjunction with formal medical treatments, there seems to be some evidence that science may be able to support its efficacy as a supplement. An early study performed by the International Society of Technology Assessment in Health care concludes with admitting there is "a strong possibility of a true metabolic effect for persons with diabetes and ingestion of prickly pear cactus." Other research supports that idea.

Not only does prickly pear have known antioxidant properties, it contains both valuable fiber and mucilage, providing a complex carbohydrate proven to slow down glucose absorption.

Usually taken in capsule form for diabetic treatment purposes, it has long been a staple, traditional vegetable in Mexican cuisine, and can also be prepared as an infusion.

There are two parts of the plant you can eat: The pads ("nopalitos") and the pear fruit (called – curiously – "tuna" in Mexico.)

Remember – if you are planning to give this supplement to a child, always double check with a medical professional who is familiar with this supplement first! One of the biggest dangers of supplements that are effective can lie in inadvertently altering the levels or the effects of previously stable doses of regular medications.

Cinnamon

Cinnamon is a spice and herb from a tree found in India and Sri Lanka. Cinnamon has been shown to lower blood sugar levels and perhaps even fats in the bloodstream like cholesterol or triglycerides that are often also abnormally high in people with diabetes. Sprinkling good quality cinnamon on food such as a whole grain bowl of oatmeal can help control blood sugar levels.

A small study in the Diabetes Care journal showed that this pleasant spice can improve blood glucose stability in Type II patients, as well as lowering:

- LDL Cholesterol
- Cholesterol
- Fasting blood glucose levels
- Triglycerides

There have been other studies, as well as lots of anecdotal evidence, supporting this result. The American Journal of Clinical Nutrition reported a simple Swedish study involving test subjects fed daily portions of rice pudding; half with cinnamon, and half without. Results showed that those who had eaten the rice pudding with cinnamon sprinkled on top did not experience the same rise in blood sugar as those without this tasty spice.

Cinnamon can be sprinkled on desserts, or used as a "tea". It can come in cinnamon-stick form, for flavoring herb teas – but for children, the safest form is simply sprinkled on food, since any accidental overdose – possible with infusions – can cause severe side effects.

You can make a delightful homemade applesauce by cutting up organic apples and cooking them down in water with cinnamon added to either a chunky or very smooth consistency.

Cloves

There is limited evidence to show that cloves also have a mildly beneficial effect, similar to cinnamon, but this herb doesn't seem to be used very often in every day North American cooking.

You'll sometimes find it as an ingredient in herbal teas – but if you're going to bake that apple pie laced with cinnamon and sweetened with stevia, add a tiny sprinkling of ground cloves, or half a dozen whole ones, too. That's the traditional European way to make apple pie – and it does add a unique flavor.

And by the way, chewing whole cloves was a trick that young men and women used to use in Victorian days before their equivalent of a "date," to sweeten their breaths.

Ginseng (Panax Quinquefolius, Panax Ginseng)

This root is also touted as a natural remedy for diabetes, though it is not recommended for children. Ginseng has a whole list of alarming side effects and possible interactions with foods and medications.

Side effects include lowering the heart rate, causing palpitations, and elevating blood pressure. For this reason, it is best to find an experienced herbalist to tell you if ginseng even makes sense for you to try as part of your regimen.

Ginseng is reported to stabilize blood sugar, and its ginsenosides are "steroidal" in nature, with reported anti-inflammatory properties. Adult dosage levels for diabetics are generally given as 100-200 milligrams. However, even if you are an adult diabetic, discuss this supplement thoroughly with your doctor and an herbal expert before trying it.

It can interact with a variety of oral diabetes medications. People with high blood pressure report it consistently causes severe headaches.

Garlic

Though pungent, it has had reported benefits in multiple studies, in keeping blood glucose levels lower after meals. That is not its only benefit, however: It has also been observed to decrease serum cholesterol levels.

Adding fresh garlic can enhance the flavor of many different foods. Garlic powder can also serve as a seasoning to interest your taste buds if you are trying to cut down on salt to control your high blood pressure.

Onions

Yes, the lowly everyday onion is said to lower blood glucose levels, when included with meals. There have been enough studies to make it universally accepted that this effect does in fact occur – especially if one can tolerate the onions raw. Children may accept this in tasty, marinated salads.

The downside? Well, both onion and garlic do make your breath smell. But there's really nothing to cry about, when you consider the health benefits!

Fenugreek

Fenugreek is a plant herb that is found naturally in the Mediterranean area and China. This substance can lower blood sugar levels and may have a limited benefit in lowering high blood cholesterol levels as well. Sometimes you can find it in tea form.

This is one of several herbs that pregnant or nursing women should not use — so again, talking with your doctor about your personal situation before trying any herb is very important.

Bilberry

Bilberry is the European blueberry. This herb is well known for its benefits on improving eyesight, but it also has the ability to lower blood sugar that is elevated. Herbalists recommend using this herb in a strong tea made from the leaves of the plant. It can take several cups of bilberry to lower blood sugar, but again, this can vary from person to person.

Herbs for External Injuries and Wounds

Wounds or injuries in persons with diabetes or chronically high blood sugar levels can be very dangerous. Particularly in diabetics whose blood sugars are high, the body loses many important nutrients that is normally uses in the fight against infections.

Without early treatment, seemingly minor infections in the extremities can lead to the spread of the infection in the body and amputations. But, good blood sugar control and a strong preventive nutritional program can significantly reduce these risks.

Some of these nutrients include the **mineral zinc and vitamin C**. The high blood sugar levels often lead over time to impaired wound healing and nerve damage, making a diabetic less likely to even realize they even have an injured or infected toe or a foot until it is late in the damage — because the nerves that carry pain signals back to the brain no longer work properly.

As a result, it is extremely important to have your doctor look at any significant injury or wound if you are diabetic (or even if you are not). Do good first aid, regardless – apply pressure to stop bleeding, wash the wound with running water if possible to knock out as many bacteria as possible too.

Avoid using a tourniquet, which will reduce blood flow to the body part. Hydogen peroxide may help wash out dirt from a deep wound, but it may also damage surrounding skin – so be careful.

You can often talk with a nurse at your health insurance company or an urgent care center about immediate steps to take that are best for your particular situation.

Don't try to self treat any injury that is more than a minor cut or burn. Deep wounds also need professional evaluation and treatment, as well as a tetanus shot or booster to avoid a very serious infection that can occur.

For minor wounds and cuts, you can find external healing salves and ointments such **as Calendula gel or Comfrey salves** (Never take Comfrey internally – it can be toxic). Other external home remedies for minor cuts include garlic juice, rosemary, and goldenseal applied to the injured area. Any gaping wound needs medical attention, not home remedies.

Nonetheless, there are some other home remedies or natural remedies for healing wounds that may help the healing process.

First, make sure that you take a good supplement of zinc and of vitamin C – you may even be able to get some lozenges usually used for colds to get the amounts you need internally. Don't overdo the zinc – it needs to be in balance with copper, but both are needed for cells to heal well. Make sure your diet includes good quality protein.

Not only is protein good to help control blood sugar in pre diabetes and diabetes, it also is essential to help the inflammatory and immune response processes to occur properly and assist new tissue to grow and fill in the wound.

Next, scientists have been finding that while some honey may have bacterial contamination, honey applied outside the body to a wound naturally has antibiotic properties. Honeys differ in which ones work better, but overall, when it is OK to block dirt and air from the wound, **Manuka honey** can do so and kill bacteria that try to grow in the injured area.

In addition, honey may have some anti-inflammatory properties, along with some ability to reduce pain. Obviously, if you are allergic to honey or to bees, this is not a strategy for you.

Another alternative for external application with antibacterial and antifungal effects is salves or lotions containing **tea tree oil** (it must be diluted in something else, often almond oil and beeswax or some other material, as it is too concentrated for direct application on its own).

Apple cider vinegar is another home remedy to promote natural wound healing. The vinegar may have some ability to blocking itching as the wound begins to heal. It may not be the first thing to put on a wound right after an injury, but it may help later in the course of healing when the itching becomes more difficult to deal with.

Other natural substances with antibiotic properties include **colloidal silver** oro grapefruit seed extract (diluted) in a spray externally, or, as noted above, diluted tea tree oil (which has antibiotic and antifungal properties).

External vitamin E creams sometimes can help reduce scarring when the wound is finishing up its healing.

Again, always make sure that your doctor monitors what you are doing so that everything you do works together and helps the wound healing along, especially if you are prediabetic or diabetic with elevated blood sugar levels.

Hibiscus Can Significantly Lower Blood Pressure in Diabetics

Hibiscus tea is made from the infusion of the sepals or calyces of Hibiscus sabdariffa flower. It is an herbal tea drink that can be consumed either hot or cold by people from all over the world. It has a cranberry-like, tart flavor and sugar can be added as a sweetener to the beverage.

It contains decent levels of vitamin C and other minerals and is a traditional form of medicine.

It contains about 15 − 30% of organic acids which includes tartaric acid, maleic acid and citric acid. It also consists of flavonoid glycosides like delphinidin and cyaniding, as well as acidic polysaccharides where its deep red color is from.

Hibiscus tea daily

High blood pressure is a common problem that people with high blood sugar also face. Blood pressure can be significantly reduced among people who drink hibiscus tea daily. For these people with elevated risks of kidney or cardiovascular disease, two to three cups of this promising herb may just be the answer.

According to new findings that were presented at an annual conference for the American Heart Association, people with high blood pressure can benefit greatly from drinking this fragrant tea. High blood pressure is frequently a problem that people with type 2 diabetes also experience, and it can markedly increase the risk of heart attack and stroke.

Related research study

McKay and colleagues studied 65 individuals who ranged from the ages of 30 up to 70 years old. Their high blood pressure levels put them at risk for having a heart attack, kidney disease, and stroke. These participants were asked to drink either a placebo tea or hibiscus tea three times in a day for a total of six weeks.

By the end of the study, their blood pressure had fallen at an average of 7.2% in the group drinking hibiscus tea as compared to only 1.3% with the placebo group. The reduction in the hibiscus group reached as much as 13.2% in some participants.

A promising natural remedy

Hibiscus is now considered as one of the most promising herbal medicines for the treatment of blood pressure. The studies showed that individuals who consume two cups of

86

hibiscus tea every day for at least four weeks had lowered their blood pressure by at least 12 %. These results are almost as good as those of commonly used blood pressure medications. But, those drugs can increase your risk of diabetes and have many uncomfortable side effects.

Improves blood vessel functions

Scientists are not entirely sure which compounds in the hibiscus flower contribute to the protective effect, but it is known that these flowers have chemicals called anthocyanins that can improve and optimize blood vessel functioning.

They also strengthen and protect the collagen protein, which in turn gives structure to tissues, cells and blood vessels. These anthocyanins as well as other hibiscus tea components are said to be antioxidants that can cleanse the body of harmful free radicals. Free radical damage to cells is linked to cancer, symptoms of aging and heart disease.

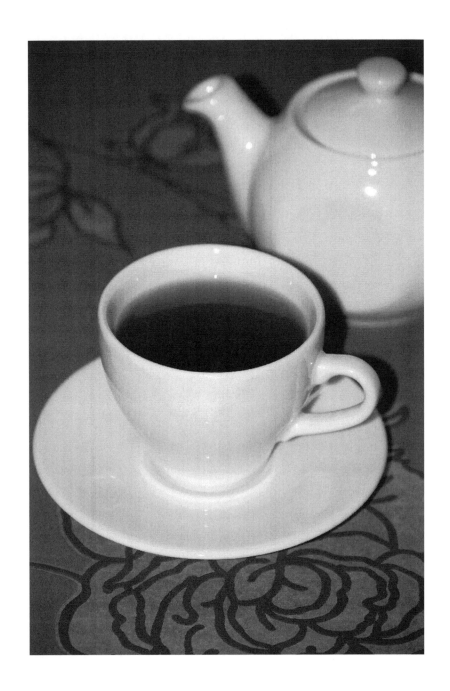

Vitamins, Minerals, and Antioxidants for Diabetes

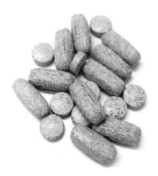

Elevating the Lowly Multivitamin

It turns out to be very important for anyone with diabetes or high blood sugar levels to take a good multivitamin and multimineral supplement.

Apart from variations in the quality of your diet, research has shown that this simple step can reduce colds and other upper respiratory infections in people with diabetes. In turn, having fewer colds or even less severe colds will help improve blood sugar control, since infections release immune system mediators that can increase insulin resistance and raise blood sugar levels (see the Appendix for more guidelines on sick day management of elevated blood sugars).

The Link Between Vitamin D and Diabetes

Recent studies showed that Vitamin D deficiency may put people to a higher risk of developing both type 1 and 2 diabetes. Although no direct link can be found between Vitamin D and diabetes, the results of these findings are impressive.

Let's have a look at this research. In a study of more than 5,000 people, researchers found that those with lower Vitamin D levels had a 57% increased risk of developing type 2 diabetes compared to people with Vitamin D levels within the desirable range.

The study also suggested that blood levels of Vitamin D higher than what is recommended for bone health may be necessary to reduce the risk of developing type 2 diabetes. It may be interesting to note that "receptors to both type 1 and 2 diabetes for its activated form-one alpha twenty-five dihydroxy Vitamin D3, have been identified in beta cells and immune cells."

In medical terms, Vitamin D deficiency has been shown to impair insulin synthesis and secretion in humans and in animal models of diabetes, suggesting a role in the development of type 2 diabetes. Diabetes risk may be higher in northern areas of the world where sunlight is not as strong for many months of the year.

The body can synthesize large amounts of vitamin D in the skin, but you have to allow direct exposure of your skin to the sunlight for this natural process to occur. Most people spend 90% of their days indoors, and many wear sunscreens that block the ultraviolent rays necessary to trigger skin synthesis of vitamin D. For these reasons, taking supplements and getting your blood levels of vitamin D checked are pragmatic steps to take.

Can delay diabetes onset

To be more explicit, researchers say that 1-alpha-25 dihydroxy vitamin D3 or its structural analogues have been shown to delay the onset of diabetes, mainly through immune modulation. They further reported that Vitamin D deficiency may be involved in causing both types of diabetes, and a better understanding of the mechanism involved, could lead to the development of preventive strategies.

In a study of Australian adults, scientists discovered that "lower levels of Vitamin D circulating in the blood stream may lead to a higher risk of developing diabetes." Obviously, all these studies point to one thing. There appears to be a link between Vitamin D deficiency and diabetes.

How high levels of Vitamin D work to lower the risk of developing diabetes has yet to be established. Experts are currently debating the proper amounts for supplements and the optimal blood levels to achieve. Some are satisfied with blood levels just above 30 ng/ml, where others insist that ideal blood levels for vitamin D are 50-70 ng/ml. It is believed that toxicity can occur above blood levels of 100 ng/ml.

Experts appear to agree that levels below 20 ng/ml are deficient, and that vitamin D deficiency is epidemic in the U.S. and other developed nations, with a rate of 41.6% of the adult population, especially in obese individuals. The Vitamin D deficiency problem is even more severe for African-Americans and Hispanics, an interesting correlation, given the higher rates of diabetes in these two groups.

Take adequate supply

It makes sense for you as a prediabetic or diabetic to make sure that you have an adequate supply of Vitamin D in your system. It is therefore important to know some basic facts of Vitamin D and how to acquire sufficient supply of Vitamin D.

As already discussed, vitamin D is produced by the body in response to skin exposure to the sun. However, it can also be found in its natural form in some food, like eggs, cod and salmon.

The best known fact about Vitamin D is its "working relationship" with calcium in building bones. The Institute of Medicine recommends that adults should have about six hundred IU of Vitamin D daily "to maintain circulating levels within the desired range."

Other experts focus on the amount of supplementation needed to achieve a particular blood level, and then the recomended amounts vary widely. Some claim that people can need 3,000 to 5,000 IU per day or more to get their blood levels into a good range. Since your doctor can do a simple blood test and find out your status, this is a good starting point for titrating the amount of supplementation you as an individual might need.

Helps control blood sugar levels

Just to show how beneficial Vitamin D is, it has also been found that Vitamin D may also help bring blood sugar levels under control. This is important considering that in type 2 diabetes; the body can't get the cells to respond properly to insulin and maintain lower blood sugar levels.

Vitamin D may have a role in increasing the release of insulin, or at least, in lessening insulin resistance. Overall, there is no doubt that Vitamin D plays an important role in reducing the risk of developing diabetes and potentially reducing the need for blood sugar drugs.

What we know of as "vitamin D" is actually composed of two fat-soluble components: vitamin D2 (ergocalciferol) and vitamin D3 (cholecalciferol). The D3 form is the more active, and some people may have metabolic problems converting D2 into D3. Therefore, it is vital for you to read the label of your supplements to make sure that you get an adequate amount of the D3 form.

Vitamin D performs a variety of tasks to help humans keep healthy, but specific to diabetes, it is implicated in modulating immune function, as well as neuromuscular function, and reducing inflammation. Some doctors claim that vitamin D can reduce the risk of getting the flu or other respiratory infections.

Since vitamin A, which co-occurs in some vitamin D cod liver oil supplements, can be toxic if upper limits are exceeded, be extra careful to follow the recommended dosages -- and double check with your medical professional before using.

It is very possible to find supplemental sources of vitamin D3 alone. A good preparation might suspend the vitamin in olive oil, as this is a fat-soluble vitamin that benefits from a carrier that is itself a fat.

During the summer, a healthy, balanced diet and outdoor activities may be all that is needed. However, in winter, when sunlight is minimal, vitamin D supplementation may be necessary – and not only for people with diabetes.

Magnesium

Magnesium is an essential dietary mineral. It occurs in higher amounts in:
- Leafy Greens
- Nuts
- Seeds
- Whole Grains
- Barley

One of its most important functions is to regulate blood sugar. It also helps maintain healthy nerve function, immune function and muscle, and these are also areas much affected by diabetes. It works to facilitate literally hundreds of enzymes, including those specific to blood glucose and insulin secretion.

If you suffer from insomnia or legs cramps at night, low magnesium could be contributing (of course, other minerals can play a role too -- low levels of iron or an excess of zinc over copper can cause restless legs symptoms).

There are indications that low magnesium levels decrease blood glucose control, especially in type II diabetes. On the other hand, studies have also shown that taking magnesium can help reduce Type II diabetics' insulin resistance and lower fasting blood sugar levels.

It can be taken as a supplement. Note, however, that high doses can cause unpleasant and severe side effects, including:

- Anorexia
- Breathing difficulty
- Diarrhea
- Irregular heart rhythm
- Low Blood Pressure
- Muscle weakness
- Nausea

Ideally, experts suggest that you take a ratio of approximately 2:1 calcium to magnesium supplementation to get the amounts of both minerals that you need. For many adults, the average amounts might then be 1,000 mg calcium and 500 mg magnesium per day.

Chromium

The most amazing discovery about chromium picolinate and diabetes is the simple fact that it can help with everything from type II diabetes to the totally unpredictable gestational diabetes. What researchers have found is that all types of insulin resistance, whether temporary or severe, will respond well to the use of this seemingly miraculous mineral.

Unfortunately, most diabetics are at risk for developing further health problems, such as heart disease, and this too leads to more dependence on pharmaceutical compounds. Many of these drugs cause the body to become depleted of all kinds of minerals and other nutrients, including essential vitamins and chromium.

This means that any of the benefits that these compounds might provide in the fight against diabetes is dramatically reduced because of the drug side effects. When you as a diabetic supplement your daily diet with higher amounts of chromium picolinate, however, you are more likely to experience a substantial and measurable decline in diabetes symptoms.

What studies are demonstrating is that it requires a higher dosage to have the best effects. For example, 200 mcg of chromium three times per day is the level that generated the best results in patients struggling to control diabetes. This amount actually lowered glucose levels even though most of the studies also simultaneously reduced the use of pharmaceutical oral hypoglycemic drugs by 50%.

The evidence from lab studies is compelling – chromium picolinate is part of the solution for those with type 2 diabetes. But as with any supplement, it is essential to discuss its use with your doctor.

Chromium works to improve your body's digestion of fat and carbohydrates. This helps your body's cells to respond to insulin in a normal, healthy way. Those who have low chromium levels often have prediabetes.

Zinc

Add zinc to your diet and/or take a supplement that includes this mineral. Zinc helps to work in the production of insulin and helps your body to store it properly. Many people with high blood sugar lose too much zinc in their urine and have increased trouble healing cuts and injuries as a result.

To make sure you have enough (but not too much), taking a supplement with the recommended daily allowance for your age is a wise move.

In its role of supporting healthy immune function, zinc may also help you fight off an incipient sore throat or cold a little faster.

Vanadium

Vanadium is a trace mineral that is found in most plants and animals. It is largely not well understood, but it appears in pharmacological doses to act in an insulin-like manner in lowering blood sugar.

As with any trace mineral, there are risks of overdoing the dose. Given the more limited experience in managing it in diabetics, it may be preferable to work with the other, better studied minerals first.

However, some alternative medicine doctors give vanadium supplements to their difficult-to-treat diabetes patients. In addition, if you are someone with osteoporosis (thinning of the bones, common in older persons, especially postmenopausal women), vanadium may also help rebuild bone mass.

Whenever you can find a supplement to do multiple good tasks at the same time, it may be worth a closer look.

Alpha Lipoic Acid

Alpha lipoic acid is a versatile antioxidant that can help in the treatment of diabetes and diabetic neuropathy. As diabetes progresses, especially when blood sugar is poorly controlled, many areas of the body are damaged, including peripheral nerves. Eventually, the nerve damage can lead to chronic pain in feet and/or hands. The usual way that doctors treat the pain is symptomatic — that is, they will try drugs from different classes such as antidepressants, antiseizure medications, or major analgesic drugs like opiates.

The trouble is, the drugs lessen the pain for many people with diabetes, but they are not able to treat the underlying disease process or the progression of the nerve damage. Researchers have found that alpha lipoic acid, a natural antioxidant substance that can recycle other antioxidants like vitamin C or vitamin E, reduces diabetic neuropathy pain. Lipoic acid can also lessen insulin resistance and help lower elevated blood sugar levels.

A recent review of multiple large studies on 1,160 patients, testing the effects of lipoic acid for diabetic neuropathy (they call it polyneuropathy because more than one nerve is usually damaged) found that it helps.

The studies used lipoic acid either intravenously at a dose of 600 milligrams per day for 3 weeks or by mouth up to 5 weeks. Patients tolerated the treatment well without major side effect problems (Mcllduff and Rutkove, *Ther Clin Risk Manag* 2011; 7:377-85). Multiple studies support the potential value of lipoic acid in diabetics.

Another benefit of lipoic acid is that it is both fat- and water-soluble. It can apparently also protect the brain from episodes of low oxygen or low blood sugar or other short-term insults, at least in animals. It even may improve memory in older animals. It is not clear if it has these types of benefits for people, but it seems to be a very worthwhile supplement to consider adding to your daily regimen.

Other research has found that people can experience nausea or even vomiting as one of the more likely side effects. To minimize this problem, dissolving the capsules in a fruit smoothie with perhaps some protein powder might help, or at least taking the supplement after food.

Test different brands of lipoic acid, as some may have a formulation that works better for you. Some report that for oral use (you can buy it in a health food store), the *R form that is well stabilized* is the best way to take lipoic acid.

You can always start with a lower dose and work your way up. Watch your blood sugar along the way – it is very possible that it will reduce your need for diabetic hypoglycemic oral drugs or insulin. That can become dangerous if you are not monitoring your blood sugar often enough when you first start using the lipoic acid.

Finally, there are rare risks of serious adverse events, but early research reported that animals who were deficient in vitamin B1 or thiamine sometimes died when taking alpha lipoic acid supplementation.

This is only possibly relevant to someone who is a severe alcoholic, as they deplete their B complex vitamins including thiamine and folic acid. Supplementation with a good B complex vitamin before starting alpha lipoic acid should help offset some of the brain and nerve damage that the alcohol itself can cause anyway.

Bottom line- it is worth a try to see if lipoic acid can help you if you are diabetic and need treatment for neuropathy (peripheral nerve pain) affecting your hands or feet. Always discuss this first with your own health care provider so that they can monitor your progress and adjust your meds if needed.

It is always a bit risky to assume that what researchers learn from rats and mice can apply to human beings and their blood sugar levels. But, many discoveries about health begin with laboratory studies in animals.

A recent study of the super antioxidant resveratrol is worth a look, even though it was done on lab rats. The press release from the investigators tells us that exposure to this natural antioxidant in young rats after weaning later prevents the development of what is called "metabolic syndrome."

Metabolic syndrome is the set of health problems leading up to the development of type 2 diabetes, the most common and spreading form of diabetes. High blood sugar levels, partly from resistance of the body cells to the normal effects of the pancreatic hormone insulin to take up and use glucose properly, is a major part of this condition.

Here is what the press release specifically says:
"Resveratrol is found in fruits, nuts and red wine, and has been shown to extend the lifespan of many species.

Human offspring that have trouble growing in the womb have an increased risk of developing metabolic problems later in life. But U of A medical researchers Jason Dyck and Sandra Davidge and their teams found that administering resveratrol to the young offspring of lab rats after weaning actually prevented the development of a metabolic syndrome, which is characterized by glucose intolerance, insulin resistance and higher deposits of abdominal fat.

Dyck and Davidge published their findings in a recent edition of the peer-reviewed journal *Diabetes*. Dyck is a researcher in the departments of Pediatrics and Pharmacology, while Davidge is a researcher in the departments of Obstetrics & Gynecology and Physiology. Both are also members of the Mazankowski Alberta Heart Institute, as well as the Women and Children's Health Research Institute. Dyck and Davidge were co-senior authors of the study.

The study took advantage of the fact that "infancy is a potential window of opportunity to intervene and prevent the future development of metabolic diseases." The researchers noted this is the first potential pharmacological treatment that may help babies that developed in a growth-restricted environment in the womb.

"There is a concept that in utero, there are genetic shifts that are occurring – reprogramming is occurring because of this strenuous environment babies are in, that allows them to recover very quickly after birth," says Dyck.

"When babies are growth-restricted, they usually have a catch-up period after they are born where they catch up to non-growth-restricted groups. It might be that reprogramming that creates this kind of 'thrifty' phenotype, where they want to consume and store and get caught up.

"That reprogramming appears to make them more vulnerable to developing a host of metabolic problems."

Earlier this year, Dyck and Davidge published another paper in *Diabetes* demonstrating that rat offspring not growing well in the womb had noticeable side effects from high-fat diets after birth – the rats deposited more fat in the abdominal area, developed glucose intolerance, more dramatic cases of insulin resistance and insulin resistance at earlier stages of life.

Also, other research has shown that eating higher quality proteins with all of the essential amino acids in adequate amounts and balance can also contribute to less belly fat accumulation. Your diet really does matter.

Dyck and Davidge are continuing their research in this area, examining whether treating the mother during pregnancy can prevent metabolic problems in rat offspring affected by intrauterine growth restriction."

GABA

The epidemic of type 2 diabetes in the U.S. and around the world has increased focus on finding ways to lower insulin resistance and convince the body's cells to take up glucose from the blood more normally.

Many people also have trouble tolerating medications or are just afraid of the long term risks of some of these meds (such as rosiglitazone). Or the meds just don't work, and the person with type 2 diabetes faces adding insulin to batter the cells into submission to accept glucose from the bloodstream.

Any natural remedy that might help avoid adding insulin and/or reduce the amount of diabetes drugs needed is a potentially welcome discovery. In an animal study, researchers may have found another such dietary supplement to consider – GABA or gamma-aminobutyric acid.

GABA is usually better known as the neurotransmitter in the brain that calms down nerve firing to reduce insomnia and anxiety. It is not even clear if GABA in this study got into the brain – it may just be acting outside the brain.

It is possible that the GABA acts by helping to inhibit inflammation and/or reduce hypertension. Any kind of chronic inflammation in the body can increase insulin resistance and reduce glucose tolerance.

One strategy for thinking about how to put together a unique program of natural remedies is to know how each one of the supplements might work on insulin resistance.

Hitting the problem from all sides might be more helpful to promote blood sugar health than going only at the problem from one direction, such as trying to add even more insulin.

Coenzyme Q10 and Diabetes

Coenzyme Q10 is defined as a naturally occurring compound found in every cell in the body especially in the heart, liver, kidneys and pancreas and helps convert food into energy. It is produced by the body and is necessary for the basic functioning of cells. Coenzyme Q10 is eaten in small amounts and is found in meats and sea food. As we age, we probably need more CoQ10 than we can get from diet alone.

There are conflicting results on studies concerning Coenzyme Q10's health benefits for diabetes. When scientists disagree, it is often the details of the study designs that can help you understand why.

For example, with CoQ10, some people's metabolism is not as good as others in converting CoQ10 into the biologically most active form. So, if a study used a less active form or a lower dose than another study, the results could turn out different. So, for your purposes, as with many natural supplements, look for the more active form of CoQ10, ubiquinol, to see if it really can help you.

No effect on glycemic control?

Coenzyme Q10 daily, 200 mg per day of fenofibrate (a lipid regulating drug), both or none at all were studied for twelve weeks. Patients with coenzyme Q10 supplementation had significantly improved blood pressure and glycemic control. However, two other studies showed that coenzyme Q10 supplementation did not have any effect on blood sugar control or levels.

Nonetheless, the positive effects of Coenzyme Q10 on alleviating heart disease, kidney failure, high blood pressure and other diseases cannot be overemphasized.

Perhaps in the not too distant future, more extensive research and studies can provide a more conclusive answer, if not a link, between coenzyme Q10 and diabetes.

In the meantime, if you are on statin drugs to lower cholesterol, like many diabetics, you need a CoQ10 supplement to prevent the drug itself from depleting your Coenzyme Q10 levels, making your muscles weak and turning your quality of life in a bad direction.

Positive response to coenzyme Q10

Note that various diseases which may be considered as an offshoot of diabetes are known to have responded positively to coenzyme Q10, Complications resulting from diabetes include cardiovascular diseases such as cardiac arrests, congestive heart failure, hypertension, and kidney failure. The possibility that there is indeed a link between low levels of coenzyme Q10 and diabetic complications needs to be further explored.

Coenzyme Q10 produces energy for the body, and functions as a vitamin-like substance found in every cell of the human body. It's other name, ubiquinone, is related to the root word "ubiquitous," which means "found everywhere". This alone emphasizes the vital role that coenzyme Q10 plays in the human body. Just for its effects on heart health alone for you as a diabetic or pre diabetic, it is worth adding to a daily regimen of natural supplements.

Some animal research suggests that low CoQ10 may contribute to kidney disease complications of diabetes, and CoQ10 may help reverse this problem. Other animal studies have shown that Coenzyme Q10 supplements may protect the liver from free radical damage (oxidative stress) and inflammation caused by obesity from a high-fructose diet. Fructose is a common sugar added to sodas and a big factor in weight gain.

Bottom Line: CoQ10 benefits for diabetics

Think of the benefits to the health and well-being of diabetics once this link is established, considering the fact that coenzyme Q10 is found in every cell of the human body, especially in vital organs like the heart, liver, and kidney. Its ubiquitous presence in the body provides the key that could unlock the enormous potential of coenzyme Q10 as a protective remedy against major complications in type 2 diabetes.

Your Action Steps:

1. Ask your doctor about trying nutritional supplements to add to your current treatment program for high blood sugar.

Focus on the specific vitamins and minerals discussed in this chapter.

2. If you have nerve damage and pain in your extremities from excessively high blood sugars, ask about a trial of R-alpha lipoic acid (by mouth) for 2-3 months.

3. Be patient. Nutritional supplements are natural and take time to act within your body chemistry.

That means vitamins and minerals are not drugs and they do not usually slam your body into submission the way some drugs do. Allow at least 3 months, perhaps even 6 months, to evaluate the full benefits or lack of benefits from adding nutritional supplements.

Stress Relief for Blood Sugar Control

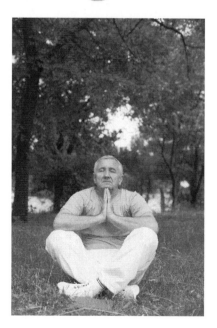

Stress is a regular experience in our lives, like it or not. To keep stress from causing health problems for you, there are a number of different non-drug techniques and alternative therapies that you can add to your total package of self-care.

For diabetics, this is especially important. The stress hormones and sympathetic nervous system activity that you mo bilize when you react adversely to stress will raise your blood sugar (and, often, your blood pressure).

While you might not be able to avoid all stress, you can take steps to relieve stress when you feel as though you're under pressure. With these stress relief tips for diabetics, you can feel calm and collected, even in the most stressful times.

- Exercise regularly – One of the best ways to relieve your stress is to exercise regularly. When you exercise, your body releases feel-good hormones and the more you exercise, the better you feel. Try to exercise for at least thirty minutes a day for the best results.

- Socialize – Getting together with your friends and family on a regular basis will help you to relieve your stress as well. Try to go out with those you love at least a few times a month to ensure you're not isolating yourself and your stress.

- Take time for yourself – Because you might have a number of responsibilities in your life which could cause stress, it's a good idea to make sure you're taking some time for yourself, doing things that you want to do without anyone else around.

- Meditate – Taking just 10 minutes a day to sit in a quiet space will allow your brain to learn the skill of emptying the stressful feelings. Close your eyes and sit in a comfortable place. Breathe regularly as you try to keep your brain free from extra thoughts. Even if a thought comes into your mind, just let it go. The more you practice this skill, the better you will become at reducing your overall stress levels.

- Vent – When you are angry or upset, find someone to talk to, or write in a journal to get your feelings out. If you hold onto your feelings for too long, it can cause you to feel even more stressed and less in control of your life.

- Pursue your interests – If you're interested in learning a new language or a new skill, get out and find a way to learn more about your interests. The more that you pursue your interests, the more you will have something about which to be excited, which will help to reduce your overall feeling of stress.

As a diabetic, it's crucial that you manage your diet, but you also need to regulate the amount of stress you feel so that you're not reaching for foods that undermine your needs and your health. Remember that stress is a part of your life, but it does not need to be something that controls your attitude and your mental state. You can overcome your stress when you relieve it, instead of letting it build up.

Here are some outstanding alternative therapies that can help you control stress and promote a better sense of well-being and energy in yourself with regular use...

Yoga for Diabetics

Diabetics need to focus not only on managing their blood sugar levels, but also their stress levels. With a proper stress relief program, you will be able to ensure your body is not suffering from undue stress. Yoga is one practice that will help to support your body with activity, while also helping to lower your body's reaction to stressful feelings and situations.

Yoga is an ancient Hindu practice from India used worldwide for health promotion and stress reduction. It is one of a number of drug alternative approaches to lowering blood sugar levels in people who are pre diabetic or diabetic.

A 3-month study of yoga for people with the most common form of diabetes, Type 2, in which blood sugar levels are often extremely high, shows that yoga can help lower blood sugar and improve other measures of health.

In specific, this study of 123 diabetics demonstrated not only that blood sugar control was better, but the yoga-treated individuals also lost some weight (lower body mass index or BMI) and improved in several blood tests for oxidative stress.

Oxidative stress is a by-product of metabolism in the body that can produce cell-damaging free radicals, accelerate aging and cause complications of diabetes.

There are many forms of yoga that you can start to learn. Some programs are even set up specifically for older people and people with physical disabilities. So, while you may think of very strenuous postures that you may see in people practicing yoga, these are not the whole story.

The yoga program for elders is called "Silver Yoga" or "Chair Yoga" and is very gentle and easy to learn. Yoga, like other health promoting practices, does not require any particular religious or spiritual belief, nor does it impose any ideas on you that are contrary to your own be-liefs. Rather, used in a secular way, yoga simply promotes re-balancing of the body and your energy to allow the body to unwind from stress and change the demands on your body.

Stress Relief

While you may already know that yoga is beneficial for those who have stress, some people may not know why. When you practice yoga, you're going to be moving your body into a series of postures, which will cause your brain to be focused on those activities instead of on other busy thoughts in your mind that make you tense and activate stress hormones.

In addition, you will learn how to focus your breath dur-ing harder poses, helping to train your body to release tension in your muscles and get more intense stretches. Plus, many people find yoga to have a meditative quality, which will allow them to clear their minds of stressful thoughts.

How to Learn Yoga

In order to practice yoga, you have a number of different avenues to take. Ideally, taking a class from a certified and experienced teacher is the best possible method, but you can also seek out other sources of information.

- Take classes – As with any new exercise, it's best to take classes with an instructor, especially if you haven't tried yoga before. They can work with you to place your body in the proper position.

- Use videos – Videos can help you learn more advanced positions, without having to travel to a class.

- Seek out a partner – You might also want to learn yoga with a friend who is also learning, or you could connect with a friend who already knows yoga. They can help to give you advice and move your body in the right directions.

As with anything, yoga is something that you practice and enjoy, not something that you have to be perfect at doing, right at the start.

Safe Yoga Tips

To make sure that yoga is helping you as a diabetic, as well as helping your body, make sure to follow these tips:

- Move slowly – When you're going yoga, make sure that you are moving slowly from position to position, especially at first. Once you know the positions, then you can begin to speed up your positions a bit.

- Don't strain – If you begin to feel a strain in your body, then stop doing what you're doing or stop stretching so far. You should never feel pain or discomfort during yoga.

- Breathe – It can also help to breathe more when you're practicing yoga, as this will help you release tension.

Yoga is a great practice for diabetics, so if you have the chance, add it to your daily routine.

Support Groups

People are social beings for the most part. Getting social support for coping with diabetes is a key part of relieving stress.

Finding diabetes support groups can seem hard at first, but there are several simple strategies for getting the social and emotional support from fellow people with diabetes that you need. Research has shown that social support can lower stress and even extend lives for people with serious diseases.

Stress is one of those things that you probably have come to take for granted, but it could literally be killing you...or at least making your life more miserable, not only from the emotions you feel, but also from the higher blood sugars and higher blood pressures that it can cause.

Feeling stressed releases stress hormones like cortisol and adrenalin or epinephrine. It activates the fight-or-flight part of your brain and nervous system to put you on edge. It helps you tense your muscles to run or fight. In primitive times, this was useful to keep you from being attacked and eaten by wild animals. But in modern life, it just leads to a cascade of undesirable outcomes. For people with diabetes, this can be particularly bad for your health.

As we said, among the steps you can take to beat stress is getting social support. Of course your partner or spouse, family members, and friends can help. But sometimes, putting all of the burden on them damages your relationships. And they are not in the same boat with you in the sense that many of them may not have diabetes or the unique challenges that you face.

So, what are your options? You can find the needed emotional support and practical tips from others living with diabetes every day, both offline in your local community and online in diabetes forums, blogs, Facebook, and other social networking sites.

Some support can even come from your pets – researchers have even found that petting your dog or cat can reduce physiological stress responses, and dog walking actually is associated with a better health profile, including lower BMI (body mass index or body weight), lower blood pressure, better blood sugar control, and better cholesterol.

On the people side of things, here are some steps to take:
1. Ask your doctor for a referral to a local diabetes educator or education center.

2. Join the online support program sponsored by the American Diabetes Association at http://Diabetes.org/DiabetesProgram for diabetics with type 2, and click on their "In My Community" link to find out what is going on with support groups in your local area.

3. Learn more about support for type 1 (juvenile) diabetics and their families at
http://www.jdrf.org/index.cfm?page_id=105564

4. Check out one of these larger diabetes self help forums:
online:

http://DLife.com

http://DiabetesSisters.com for women with diabetes

http://ChildrenWithDiabetes.com

http://DiabetesHandsFoundation.org (both English and Spanish speaking support forums)

http://DiabetesDaily.com

http://DiabetesForum.com

Look for an active forum with many members and posts – especially recent posts to make sure you haven't joined a ghost town online. Look around and "lurk," set up a vague screen ID if you are shy or unsure of how much you want to share at first, but at least check out the options.

You may be pleasantly surprised in how much sense of community, feeling understood and practical advice you might find.

If one support venue does not work out for you, keep looking.

Unfortunately, there are millions of people with diabetes out there in the world. You are not alone with this health problem -- you can find a group where it feels right and where you get what you need. Make it a priority to share and help others too – helping other people helps you feel worthwhile and valuable — and that too goes a long way toward reducing stress all by itself.

Meditation

Clearing the Mind - Easy Meditation Tips

Meditation is a great way to clear your mind of the worries and stresses of the day. If you're not familiar with this method of relaxation, you may think it's difficult. However with practice, you'll find that it's not hard at all. Research has shown that regular meditation can help reduce stress, including the chemistry of stress in the body. The benefits include lower blood sugar and lower blood pressure.

Simply put, meditation is an inner state of relaxed awareness. To achieve this contemplative state, you can simply focus your mind on your breath or on repeating a single sound or word over and over. You develop an altered state of consciousness in which you are awake, but peaceful.

Starting a Meditative Practice

Want to know what the hardest part of meditation is? Here's a hint: It has nothing to do with meditation at all!

The hardest part is simply *making the time to meditate.* Once you believe in its power and see its results, *you won't let anything get in the way of you and your peaceful practice.* It might be tough in the beginning, but stay with it! It'll be well worth the effort.

Make a goal for yourself and evaluate your progress as you go. **Commit to at least weekly meditations for four weeks.** After this time, evaluate whether the meditation has made a positive difference your life.

These meditation tips will help you in your quest for obtaining inner peace:

1. **Choose a time to meditate.** Find a good time for you to meditate. You can start with shorter sessions in the beginning, but generally you should shoot for between 30 minutes to an hour during each session.

116

Right when you get up or before you go to bed are good times to practice.

- *Make meditation a priority for yourself* just like you would for everything else that's important in your life.

2. **Keep an elevated posture.** If you slouch, you won't be in a good position for meditation and you're more likely to feel like falling asleep. Elevate your posture and you'll feel more open to the world. Relax in a crossed legged or other comfortable sitting position and rest your hands in your lap.

3. **Focus on your breath.** Your main goal is to keep your attention on your breath as you breathe in and breathe out. *It may help to say a mantra (sinple word or phrase)* and visualize breathing in good energy and letting out the bad energy with each cycle.

- Breathe at a pace that's comfortable for you. Work toward deep, long breaths.

4. **Acknowledge your thoughts.** You want to remain fully present while you're meditating, and there's no doubt that thoughts are going to enter your mind while you're trying to concentrate.

- Don't be frustrated by these thoughts, but at the same time don't let thoughts take your attention completely away. Acknowledge your thoughts and then bring your focus back to your breath.

5. **Fight the urge to sleep.** Many people complain of the urge to sleep during meditation sessions, mainly because it's relaxing and you're meditating during ear-

ly morning or late evening hours. Try to remain awake with focus and good posture.

6. **Maintain your practice.** After you discover the many benefits of meditating, it will most likely become a part of you forever. You may not have time to do this every day, but it's important to keep up with regular meditation sessions.

Meditation will help you keep a peaceful perspective on life and can tell you a lot of things about your true self. You can use it to relax, motivate, or energize you, depending on your purpose for each session. As you get more experienced with meditation, a more joyful and peaceful life will be yours!

How to Sit Comfortably While Meditating

Learning to sit comfortably while meditating will help you welcome more relaxation and peace of mind into your life. If you'd like to start meditating but feel too uncomfortable to sit for long, these steps will help.

Steps to Take Between Your Meditation Sessions:

1. **Keep limber.** It's easier to sit comfortably if you work on improving your flexibility in advance. Many people use yoga to accomplish this, but any program of gentle stretching will help. Just remember to warm up first to prevent injury.

2. **Maintain a healthy body weight.** Meditating can give you one more good reason to shed any excess pounds. You may feel more comfortable while meditating if you keep physically fit.

3. **Breathe deeply.** Breathing correctly plays a major role in meditating. Make it a habit to breathe from your diaphragm so your abdomen falls and rises rather than your chest. Let the air flow through your nostrils instead of your mouth.

4. **Practice good posture.** You're more likely to practice good posture on the cushion if you keep track of it even when you're not meditating. Try to always be aware of keeping your back straight and your shoulders relaxed. Imagine you're pushing your abdomen gently toward your back so you hold it slightly tucked.

5. **Cultivate a calm mind.** You'll get more out of meditating if you try to hold onto a calm mind all day. *If you start your meditation session in a peaceful state of mind, it will be easier to get into position faster and spend more time focused on your objectives.*

Steps to Take During Your Meditation Sessions:

1. **Start gradually.** It's great if you're ready now for the full lotus position, but there's nothing wrong with making a more gradual start. *Sit in a chair if it's painful to sit on the floor.* Sit for a few minutes at a time to begin with, and then increase the time in steady gradual increments that feel OK for you.

2. **Position your body correctly.** No matter how you sit, keep your back straight and your abdomen tucked under. Pretend your head is being gently lifted by a balloon so you hold it high without straining your neck. If you use a chair, keep both feet flat on the floor. If you use a cushion, cross your legs and bring your feet toward your waist. Do not push yourself –

119

this is stress reduction, not a competition.

3. **Shift positions when you need to.** Your ability to sit still for longer periods will naturally increase with time but it's always okay to shift positions if you feel pain or stiffness. Stand up and stretch or just re-cross your legs placing the other leg on top for a while. Roll your shoulders or gently bend your head toward one shoulder at a time. This is something to do even if you sit at a desk for long periods of time during the day.

4. **Figure out what to do with your hands.** There are two options that work well: rest your hands on your knees or rest them in your lap. Any arrangement that keeps your hands supported and out of the way is fine.

5. **Hold your tongue.** As you move your focus inwards and stop talking, you may experience discomfort as you become more aware of the saliva in your mouth. One easy solution is to touch the roof of your mouth with your tongue. This naturally inhibits the flow of saliva.

6. **Lower your eyes.** If visual images distract you, try lowering your eyelids so there's just a small sliver of light before you. Keep your eyes softly focused without targeting any single object. You can even close your eyes as long as it doesn't encourage you to fall asleep.

Meditation can transform your life with spiritual insights and greater peace. Learning to sit comfortably will help you focus on your objectives without any aches and pains getting in the way.

Tai Chi for Diabetics

Tai Chi is an ancient Chinese system of slow smooth physical movements for relaxing, restoring, and maintaining good health and balance. While you might not realize the impact of stress on your health, being aware of your stress levels is even more important for diabetics. Because your health condition puts more pressure and stress on your body, you need to find ways to release the tension in your body.

Tai Chi offers you a way to focus your attention to a peaceful place, while also offering you stress relief and health support. Another benefit is reducing falls in older people, as it helps you improve your balance.

Breathing and Tai Chi

When you're practicing Tai Chi, you will learn a number of movements that are accentuated by your breath. Focus on breathing evenly and deeply as you move through the practice. Not only does this allow you to release tension in your muscles, but it will also help you to settle your mind if you've been feeling a bit scattered or stress.

Holding your breath causes you to hold onto tension, which can help heighten any stressful feelings you might have in your life.

How to Practice Tai Chi

Because Tai Chi is a popular practice today, it's easier than ever to find classes, books, and videos to instruct you. The best plan to add Tai Chi to your life is to:

- Take a class – The best way to make sure that you are following Tai Chi instruction well, it's best to take a class with a qualified instructor. They can not only teach the movements, but they can help you if you are doing something incorrectly.

- Practice with videos – Once you begin to practice with a teacher, you will understand the basics of Tai Chi. From there, you can begin to practice with Tai Chi videos as you will know how you need to move.
- Practice on your own – After you have the basics of Tai Chi, it's a good idea to practice on your own so that you can learn how your body moves and you can begin to establish a personal Tai Chi practice.
- Use books to supplement your knowledge – If you still want a challenge from your Tai Chi practice, you can look at books to learn more movements and to find out other ways to move your body for stress relief.

Tai Chi is a simple practice that is non-impact and that can be done anywhere. Once you understand the basics, you can move your body and begin to have an easier time managing your stress and your blood sugar levels.

Even if you don't become the best Tai Chi practitioner, once you understand a few movements, you can use them any time you need a way to relieve your stress. Diabetics should try to use all of the stress relieving practices they can to make sure health is the number one priority.

If you have other health problems, tai chi may help with those too – even improving your balance and preventing falls (and bone fractures) as you get older. It is a great way to start each day.

Exercise for Stress Reduction in Diabetes

Exercise - Make It Fun and Easy

Did you know that exercise can actually transform your health and give you the ability to avoid either the onset of diabetes or delay or prevent complications altogether? If you have learned that your health is at risk with pre diabetes and you could develop type 2 diabetes, now is the time to make a change.

The good news is that you can make that change easily. The first step is to simply know what your problem areas are.

For many, it is being overweight. If you are overweight, your body will have a hard time using blood sugars in the right way. The more it struggles with insulin or the lack of it, the more likely you are to go into shock or face even worse stresses including a stroke.

With pre diabetes, exercise makes it easier to avoid the onset of diabetes itself. While it is also important for you to choose a low carb, high nutrient diet and to supplement your foods with a quality multivitamin, you can improve your chances of avoiding the onset of the full blown diagsnosis of diabetes through exercise.

Make It Fun

The problem is, many people do not like to exercise. And, with pre diabetes or diabetes, exercise seems like even more work. If you are struggling and just hoping you really never have to deal with this condition, think again.

Most people who are pre diabetic will develop the condition within a matter of years, if not sooner. Most people who already have diabetes will develop complications over time, if they do not control their blood sugar properly.

Exercise is one way out. The solution is to make it fun. Here are some ideas to help you.

- Focus on physical activities that you enjoy. If you like to walk, do so. If you enjoy swimming, spend some time at the pool. Perhaps you enjoy shopping. That is a great way to get in physical exercise as long as you head to the mall and keep walking.

- Plan to exercise with others. Rather than working out on your own, do it with someone else (a friend, a personal trainer)8iszxk. You are more likely to be successful if you do your pre diabetes exercise with someone else. The social interaction will work as stamina for you. Take your dog on a walk, if you can't find a human buddy to work out with.

- Do it often. You should be doing some type of physical activity for at least 30 minutes each day, at least six days per week. But, even walking 2-3 times per week is a great start.

By doing these things, you will improve your health and boost your chances of avoiding diabetes or its complications. Exercise should be something you look for and participate in regularly so that you can heal your body and your mind.

An important safety point is to review your exercise program with your doctor. In addition to the demands of the exercise itself on your body, it is likely that exercise will cause a short term drop in your blood sugar level. If you are also taking insulin or other drugs to control blood sugar, the drop could be much lower than is safe for you.

All this means is that you have to plan ahead. Even Olympic athletes with diabetes can do very strenuous exercise. They just take precautions such as adjusting their medication doses downward and having fast acting carbohydrates available for an overly low blood sugar.

Walking to Control High Blood Sugars

If you ask any medical professional for advice about an appropriate level of exercise they would tell you that it is best to get around 30 minutes of cardiovascular training each day.

This, however, does not mean you have to go to a gym, hire a personal trainer, or take any dramatic steps. Instead, it simply means that you can go for a brisk 30 to 40 minute walk each day in order to meet the minimum requirements for good health.

What is so interesting about the benefits of such a quick burst of exercise is that it can have a tremendously higher and beneficial effect for those with diabetes. For example, when you combine walking and diabetes you can enjoy improved cardiovascular fitness, and this is of tremendous value to a diabetic.

Why is that? Adults with diabetes are at a substantially higher risk for heart disease, and by improving the general level of cardiovascular exercise and fitness; it means that you are decreasing the risks for heart disease.

Another benefit of combining walking and diabetes is that you get better control over glucose levels. For example, when you exercise it actually helps the body to absorb and utilize blood sugar. This reduces the amount of stored glucose in the blood stream, and that means that you have the ability to better regulate insulin levels.

Activity such as walking will improve circulation to your extremities, something that anyone with diabetes or high blood sugar needs.

Finally, the most substantial benefit of adding walking to your natural ways to control diabetes is that you are far more likely to get your weight under control as well. This is a major issue for those with diabetes because being overweight can make it far more challenging to control blood glucose.

When you are walking each day, watching your diet, and checking blood glucose levels in order to keep them at healthy levels you are going to enjoy a far better sense of well being.

It is a great idea to combine walking and diabetes, regardless of which type of diabetes you have. It is important to discuss your choices with your regular physician because they have to give patients a formal approval to begin any sort of regular and demanding exercise.

Only your physician will know if you need to remain aware of any special precautions, have concerns about shoes or sneakers, and whether you may require alternative medications. If you do have some health concerns it is best to walk with a partner or buddy who is aware of the situation and who can ensure that you remain safe and healthy!

8 Simple Exercise Routines to Fit into Your Busy Life

Are you thinking that you don't have time to fit exercise into your busy lifestyle? Well, think again! Here are 8 simple routines that are easy to do and - best of all - they don't take much time.

Just spend 10 minutes or less on these easy activities and a new, healthier lifestyle will be yours!

As always, be sure to check with your doctor before starting any new exercise routine.

Surely you can fit these fun, healthy activities into your busy life:

1. **Jump rope.** If you haven't tried jumping rope lately, now is the time to give this fun and invigorating exercise a try. Purchase a jump rope or fashion your own from any sturdy piece of rope. *Start slowly and gradually increase both your speed and intensity.* This heart-healthy exercise can be performed a few times a day for maximum exercise benefits.

2. **Climb stairs.** Did you know that staircase in your home or workplace is actually a mini-gym in disguise? Take advantage of this exercise opportunity whenever you have a few extra minutes to spare. *Climbing stairs builds strength and gets your heart pumping.*

   - Listen to music or an audio book while going up and down the stairs. Before you know it, you'll be looking forward to your climbing sessions!

3. **Dance to the music.** Don't be shy! Turn up your favorite music and dance with abandon! Dancing is not only fun, but it's also a terrific form of exercise. Professional dancers are more fit than many professional athletes!

4. **Bounce on a mini-trampoline.** No doubt about it. Trampolines are just plain fun! Mini-trampolines can be purchased at many chain stores, sporting goods stores, or online. Pull out your trampoline and *spend just five minutes jumping away.* You may enjoy this exercise so much that you'll increase the amount of time you have available for your exercise routine.

5. **Quick calisthenics.** Everyone has, at one time or another, practiced calisthenics. Now is the time to remember those lunges, knee bends and jumping jacks of days gone by! Finding just five minutes in your hectic day to practice one or more these calisthenics exercise routines can make a big difference in your health.

6. **Lift weights.** Many exercise routines neglect that all-important need to increase upper body strength. Lifting weights solves that problem. Depending on your size and fitness level, choose the amount of weight appropriate for you. *Start with lighter weights,* and as you spend time on a daily routine, gradually increase the amount of weight you can handle.

7. **Walk faster.** Will you be walking the dog later today? Or perhaps walking from your car into the shopping mall? *Picking up your walking speed will also increase your fitness level.* Walking of any kind is always a good thing, but walking faster enhances the exercise benefits you receive from it.

8. **Practice balance.** Part of any healthy lifestyle is having good balance. The more you practice, the easier it is to maintain balance not only in your exercise routine, but also in your daily life. Practicing balance requires only a few minutes a day and best of all, can be practiced anywhere with no special equipment.

- Stand a few feet from a wall or other supporting structure and raise one foot off the ground, placing that foot gently on your other ankle or calf. Maintain balance as long as you can. Repeat the exercise with the other foot.

- *With daily practice, you'll notice a gradual increase in the amount of time you can keep your balance.*

Your Action Steps:

1. *Select one stress reduction method that appeals to you and get started. Expand to other methods as you can.*

The point is to feel better and experience more energy – so you will start looking forward to your time outs -- your stress relief sessions. They are not just another thing to add to your day. They are for you. They are enjoyable. And they help you get more energy to face your day.

2. *Discuss a realistic activity and gradual exercise plan with your health care provider. Start with a walking program.*

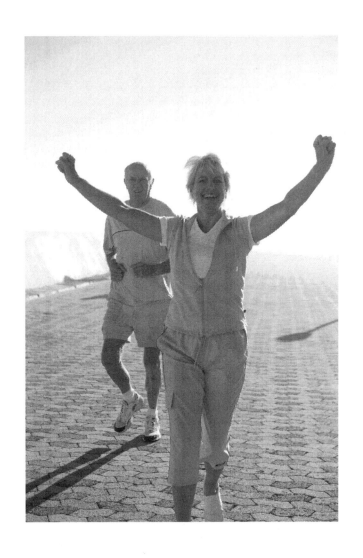

Stop Compulsive Overeating

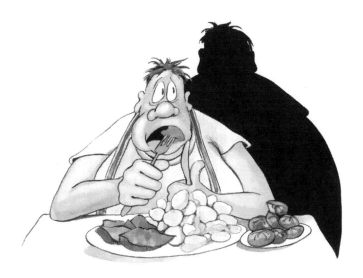

Remember when your mother cautioned you to chew your food well before swallowing it? Nutritionists tell us the importance of letting saliva start the digestive process in the mouth. And, as an adult, the mindfulness meditation experts tell us to be in the moment and experience everything, including food, as fully as possible.

Now research now reports that people who eat their food quickly have double the risk of developing pre diabetes with what is called "impaired glucose tolerance."

Even people who snack and eat food late at night do not have the same increased risk of pre diabetes that the fast eaters do.

Impaired glucose tolerance is evidence that the body is beginning to struggle with responding normally to the signals that insulin gives to cells to take up glucose (the body's fuel) from the bloodstream. As a result, the blood sugar creeps up too high. When it crosses a threshold, the person ends with the diagnosis of diabetes (type 2).

There are many other risk factors for diabetes, including being overweight or obese. Eating slowly is not necessarily a cause of the problem – it could just be a correlation. That is, the kind of person who eats fast may have other problems internally that are the real reasons behind the impaired glucose tolerance.

Still, if nothing else, people who eat fast may be stressed — and stress hormones like cortisol definitely impair glucose tolerance and foster the development of diabetes.

Still, it seems worth a try to slow down and savor your meals, bite by bite. It might help you in ways you hadn't even considered.

Hypnosis for Overeating and Weight Loss

Before you turn up your nose at the idea of weight loss hypnotherapy for diabetics you should know that many professional medical groups advocate, or at least support,

132

the idea. This is because weight loss hypnotherapy can be used as a sort of supplemental tactic for any diabetic currently following a new regimen in regards to their daily diet and exercise level.

If you do any reading about weight loss in general you will see that many experts and organizations mention the phrase "mindset" repeatedly. This is because any sort of weight loss program requires you to change the way you view everything from food and fitness to life as a whole.

Diabetics and pre diabetics who utilize weight loss hypnotherapy as a part of their new mindset will be fortifying their new attitudes and perspectives, and this can only help them to reach their goals.

How does weight loss hypnotherapy for diabetics work? Like any hypnotherapy treatment, you meet with a properly trained professional clinical hypnotist or hypnotherapist (not a stage hypnotist). Through a series of guided sessions (which can use a variety of hypnosis tactics) you will be encouraged to subconsciously shift your mindset about the way that you eat, your attitude about food, and even how you feel about fitness and exercise.

Why is this necessary? A lot of people are subconsciously sabotaging their diets as soon as they begin. For instance, consider the "forbidden factor" that often steers dieters of all kinds straight into disaster.

This is when the idea that specific foods are totally forbidden drives you to actually crave that food more and more until you "break" and go right ahead and overindulge in it. When you visit a hypnotherapist and work with them to create a strong subconscious foundation for dieting. The positive suggestions from hypnosis can reduce or eliminate this risk of falling off the wagon because of food cravings that your own mind gets obsessed about.

Let's not also overlook the simple fact that treatments of this kind often reveal certain fixations, problems, or turmoil that someone might have about food or weight loss plans too. A good hypnotist may be able to help you overcome those related challenges and succeed with your diet.

Consider that a lot of people don't recognize that they are "comfort eaters" until they begin hypnotherapy for weight loss. When such a person is also a diabetic, the benefits are going to be magnified because of the knowledge that their excess weight has health implications now. Understanding some of the underlying reasons for overeating can help you begin distinguishing hunger from boredom, upset, or sadness, and avoiding binges.

Hypnosis is a valid treatment for many conditions, and it can help a diabetic with weight loss too.

Acupuncture for Food Cravings and Overeating in Diabetes

When you're trying to manage your diabetes, there are a number of resources in conventional care. But sometimes, you might reach out for natural and alternative therapies for support in addition to your physician-prescribed program. Acupuncture is a safe and effective way to help rebalance your body's natural healing potential and to help you manage your diabetes more effectively.

What Acupuncture Does

Acupuncture is an ancient practice of placing needles at certain parts of the body in order to restore the proper

134

flow of energy throughout the body. Practitioners of acupuncture believe the body is made up of energy pathways or meridians which, if disrupted, can cause illness and other health problems. Acupuncture treatments are done over the course of a few weeks or months in order to re-stabilize your body's energy flow, and the treatments are sometimes covered by health insurance.

How Acupuncture Helps Diabetes

There are a number of purported benefits of using acupuncture for diabetes:

- Lower blood sugar
- Fewer cravings and smoother weight loss
- Increased circulation
- Better pain control without drugs
- Improved digestion

When you have an acupuncture treatment, you begin to feel more energized in mind and body, as the energy movement in your body is balanced in a more normal way. For many centuries, acupuncture, Chinese medicine, and herbs have helped others discover a better sense of well being for supporting normal blood sugar levels.

When to Use Acupuncture

Diabetic patients should always talk to their doctor first before starting any new treatment plan. This will help you ensure that any new treatments will not impact your other treatments in a negative way. Many diabetics find that using acupuncture at the same time as other treatments will be helpful, while others try to get as much benefit as they can from medical therapies first and then add acupuncture as a supportive integrative therapy.

Safety with Acupuncture

When starting an acupuncture therapy for diabetics, it's best to go to a professional who has had extensive training in working with diabetics. In addition, going to a licensed acupuncturist who uses new, sterile disposable needles for each treatment will ensure that no other health problems can occur from the treatment.

At first, it's a good idea to talk to the acupuncturist about your current diabetic treatments and what your goals for the therapy might be. They will ask you a number of questions that will then allow them to personalize your treatment and to measure your progress with each treatment. You will be pleasantly surprised to learn how many different ways acupuncture and Chinese medicine can help symptoms in many areas, from depression and anxiety to pain to indigestion to fatigue, and more.

Acupuncture is a safe alternative treatment for those who have diabetes. As with any treatment, working with your doctor and with the acupuncturist will allow you to see health benefits. Over the course of eight or more treatments, you should find that your blood sugar is easier to manage, your pain, if present, is lessened, and overall your health is gradually and gently improving. In the end, all of this may help prevent or delay any health complications that are often the result of diabetes.

"Courage is being afraid, but going on anyhow."

- Dan Rather

30 Ways To Lower High Blood Sugar: Your Cheat Sheet Summary

Some people just want a cheat sheet of steps to take to get going on lowering their blood sugar. If you are ready to go, here is a quick list, extracted for you to scan. No one tip is enough to reverse a complex problem like diabetes, but these are a good start on finding what's right for you:

1

Stop eating foods that you crave. Many people are actually "allergic" in a non-traditional way to foods that they

137

like eating too much. Common problem foods are corn (including corn sugar and syrup), wheat, yeast, milk, and eggs. Removing these foods from the diet may lower insulin resistance and improve diabetes control.

2

Take an alpha lipoic acid supplement several times a day (R-form is best). Lipoic acid can help relieve nerve pain from diabetes complications (neuropathy) as well as lower blood sugar and reduce the amount of drugs needed for diabetes management.

3

Eat meals containing fatty fish such as wild salmon at least twice per week and/or add omega-3 fish oil capsules daily to protect against heart disease by lowering triglycerides and reducing other diabetes complications.

4

Take adequate amounts of vitamin D, especially the metabolically more available form, D3 (cholecalciferol), at least 800 IU/day when you cannot be outdoors to make it on your own (from sunlight on your exposed skin). Some studies suggest that vitamin D lessens the risk of heart disease and type I diabetes. It probably improves mood and cuts down risk of getting the flu. Ask your doctor to check your blood level to be sure. You may even need 3,000-5,000 IU/day. Blood tests will tell you for sure.

5

Take a good multivitamin/multimineral supplement daily year-round, especially if you also have a chronic health condition. Diabetes can deplete nutrients from your body, and a sensible dose of a balanced multi formula may reduce your susceptibility not only to colds and flu, but also to some complications and side effects from your ongoing health issues and treatments.

6

Include a chromium supplement to improve glucose tolerance. Chromium helps the body use sugars made from foods more effectively.

7

Drink green tea (decaffeinated if you cannot tolerate too much caffeine) multiple times per day. Its constituents support healthier immune function. If you need to sweeten it, try stevia rather than sugar or artificial sweeteners.

8

Use the Peruvian herb cat's claw as a tea or herbal capsules to reduce autoimmune responses in diabetes (especially type I) and bolster immune defenses against viruses and bacteria.

9

Take magnesium supplements regularly to maintain good cardiac health and nerve function. Many diabetics lose excess magnesium in their urine as a result of high blood sugars. Magnesium can help with insomnia, anxiety, and muscle cramps in some people as an extra bonus.

10

Maintain a good intake of vitamin C to gut tolerance (diarrhea, bloating) along with vitamin E. Studies show that these antioxidant vitamins together may protect bodily tissues from the damage caused by high blood sugars in diabetes. Buffered forms of vitamin C such as calcium ascorbate may be easier on your gut than the ascorbic acid form.

11

Add grapeseed extract to other antioxidants. Grapeseed extract has specialized antioxidants and other components that can lessen damage to small capillaries (blood vessels) in the eye and kidney caused by high blood sugars in diabetes.

12

Sprinkle cinnamon on your food for its blood sugar lowering effect – as well as its pleasant flavor. Cinnamon can also lower "bad" LDL cholesterol and triglyceride levels in the bloodstream, thus also helping to reduce the risk of the cardiovascular complications.

13

Try fenugreek as an herbal seasoning on foods and/or as a tea for an additional herb that can improve glucose tolerance in some diabetics.

14

Make sure to take enough zinc in supplement form to make up for urinary losses of this and other key nutrients from high blood sugars in diabetes. Zinc is crucial to foster proper healing after injuries in diabetics.

15

Try the Ayurvedic herb gymnestra sylvestre to lower blood sugar levels. This is part of a total package of herbs and nutritional supplements that can help regulate blood sugar and reduce the amount of drugs needed for good control.

16

Get well-tolerated extract of the traditional Chinese herb bitter melon to less insulin resistance in type II diabetes. Bitter melon has effects similar to exercise on improving metabolism in muscle.

17

Adopt the traditional Mexican and Native American practice of eating prickly pear cactus products to drop blood sugar levels and even lessen cholesterol in the blood.

18

Strengthen heart function by taking coenzyme Q10 daily. Levels of Co-Q10 go down with age and various diseases, as well as common drugs such as statins. Taking Co-Q10 may slightly decrease high blood pressure and/or combat congestive heart failure from heart disease.

19

Consider taking acai berry juice, which is reported to have a low glycemic index (raises blood sugar less rapidly and/or severely than do other fruit juices). Acai may help people control appetite and lose weight, a major goal of treatment for many type II diabetics. It is not a miracle fruit, but it may be helpful.

20
Start drinking a few cups a day of chamomile tea. Researchers have shown that chamomile tea taken regularly can help reduce blood sugar levels and block the activity of certain enzymes involved in leading to diabetic complications such as nerve damage, cataracts and diabetic retinopathy in the eye, and kidney damage. Chamomile also helps calm the stress response and fosters better sleep.

21
Alternate chamomile tea with herb tea made from blueberry leaves. Europeans have used blueberry leaves to soothe gastrointestinal upsets, reduce blood sugar by over 25%, and lower triglycerides.

22
Apply homeopathic Calendula gel and/or aloe vera gel externally to speed up healing of skin areas used for testing blood sugar with fingersticks or insulin injection sites.

23
Use fennel tea daily as another natural herbal product that is caffeine-free and may lower blood sugar. Fennel also soothes the digestive system and has a sweet anise or licorice flavor that many people enjoy using with foods as a seasoning as well.

24

Put the herb tea hibiscus into your daily fluid intake plan. Three cups per day of hibiscus tea has demonstrated an ability to lower blood pressure in people with high blood pressure (hypertension), a common problem for type II diabetics.

Holistic Approaches Beyond Supplements

25

Practice simple meditation or relaxation periods once or twice a day. The evidence is excellent that taking these important time-outs from your hectic lifestyle can lower stress responses and improve outcome in a wide range of chronic health problems.

26

Improve your sense of control over your body and your life with journaling. Journaling is simply writing in a notebook or diary daily about your feelings over stressful (or pleasant) events in your life. Studies have shown that journaling leads to measurable improvements in health for people with a variety of chronic conditions.

27

Consider seeing a licensed acupuncturist or certified classical homeopath to rebalance your system. Acupuncture and homeopathy can each boost your overall sense of well-being and energy while helping your body's metabolism work in a more coordinated way. Some studies suggest that acupuncture may also even reduce depression in certain people, which is a major problem for people struggling with diabetes everyday.

28

Take a yoga class with an experienced instructor to learn an enjoyable and relaxing practice that is also drug-free and natural. Yoga may help you lower blood sugar levels, blood pressure, and weight if you have type II diabetes.

29

Learn the ancient Chinese practice of qi gong or Tai Chi for restoring and maintaining health. Some preliminary reports suggest that, like other mind-body and relaxation practices, qi gong can help lower blood sugar and improve cholesterol levels. Tai Chi helps lower stress and promote better balance

30

Take a daily walk for 45 minutes with a friend or your dog. Walking exercise is a simple, inexpensive method for improving weight loss, lowering blood sugar and "bad" fats in the blood such as LDL cholesterol and triglycerides in diabetics. Be sure to get the right walking shoes to protect your feet and then get on the move. Just standing up and not sitting for too long at a time is better for your health than doing nothing at all about physical activity.

Notice that many of the stress management strategies end up with a common theme – as in the Paul Simon song: "Slow down, you move too fast, you've got to make the morning last..."

Final Thoughts to Motivate Yourself

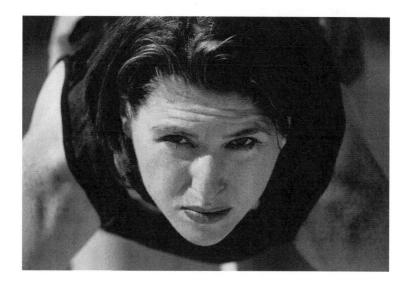

So, to sum up, here is the big picture strategy of steps for you to take to lower your blood sugar and keep it in the normal range:

1. Switch to a low carb diet *like Dr. Bernstein's Diabetes Solution* diet or another low carb diet plan. Low carb di-

ets do not always mean high fat or deprivation. They mean quality nutrition, with limited and healthier carbs.

2. Get exercise and lose some weight. There is simply no better way to avoid the development of diabetes than to cut down the weight. This gives your body a fighting chance. The good news is these diets can help you to do just that.

3. Pump up the nutrients heading into your body. You can do this easily with a multivitamin along with supplements known to actually work against pre diabetes, including cinnamon, vanadium and chromium.

4. You can also use herbs known to improve blood flow and digestions including bitter melon, gymnema and other natural treatments.

5. Find the alternative therapies that can help you deal with stress, stop compulsive overeating, and lose weight.
By using these five steps, you will transform your diet it something that is working for you and battling the problems your health is facing.

It is possible to learn how to reverse pre diabetes or diabetes. All you have to do is to pay closer attention to what your body needs. If you are obese, work on losing the weight quickly. If you eat a fatty diet, choose one of these low carb, high nutrient solutions instead. You will see results when you do.

No More Excuses - Motivate Yourself Today

You may already know that motivation is one of the keys that determine success or failure in controlling prediabetes or diabetes. However, just knowing doesn't make it any easier to gain motivation. If you feel that you're having trouble properly motivating yourself, it's time for you to act. Not tomorrow, but today.

Finding your motivation is something personal. The best way to find motivation is to explore your options and discover something that works for you.

Consider the following ways to motivate yourself today:

1. **Avoid just going through the motions.** One reason you may find it difficult to perform everyday tasks is that you get bored. Of course you're going to try to avoid something that you find tedious! You can combat this mentality by adding some depth to your thinking while you're engaging in tasks you dislike.

   - Brainstorm ways that you can complete the task in a more efficient manner. Then you can compete with yourself to see how quickly you can complete the task in the future. The quicker you get it done, the sooner you can move on to bigger and better things!

2. **Get spiritual.** Don't be afraid to get in touch with your spiritual side. Many people find it highly motivating! When you discover some answers to life's tough questions, it brings you clarity, and you may be more likely to work harder to achieve your desires.

3. **Set a goal.** You might lack motivation because you don't have a goal. If you aren't even sure what you're working towards, you'll have difficulty finding motivation.

   - If you have a large goal, ***break up the goal into a series of small, achievable tasks*** and set

147

each task as a separate goal. This helps you maintain motivation because you're constantly achieving your goals. You can *see* the results of your hard work!

4. **Hold yourself accountable.** In order to ensure that you don't stray from your chosen path, evaluate your progress every week or even every day. Determine how you can do better the next week.

   - If you find that it's difficult to keep yourself accountable, ***don't be afraid to ask for help.*** You may enjoy having others check up on you to make sure you stay on task.

5. **Think positive thoughts.** Negative thinking and lack of motivation go hand in hand. You can increase your motivation by concentrating on eliminating your negative thinking patterns. Replace negative feelings with optimism and positive thoughts and images.

   - When you catch yourself feeling down, make an extra effort to seek the silver lining. It's always there. If you take the time to look hard enough, you'll find it.

6. **Make a change.** If you think you've tried everything and you still can't get motivated, perhaps you should consider a life change. Maybe there's a reason why you're feeling this way. If depression is part ofo the problem, get help from your doctor or a therapist.

   - If you don't feel motivated to work toward your major life goals, consider some alternatives that may be more in line with your true desires.

- If you're having trouble finding motivation for everyday chores, see if you can find a way to hire some help.

Always keep in mind that "the time is now." Put procrastination into your past and you'll feel happy and accomplished at the end of the day, instead of stressed out or regretful.

When you're motivated, life is more fulfilling. Use these strategies to wake up your motivation and enjoy the difference!

"The greatest mistake you can make in life is to be continually fearing you will make one."

-- Elbert Hubbard

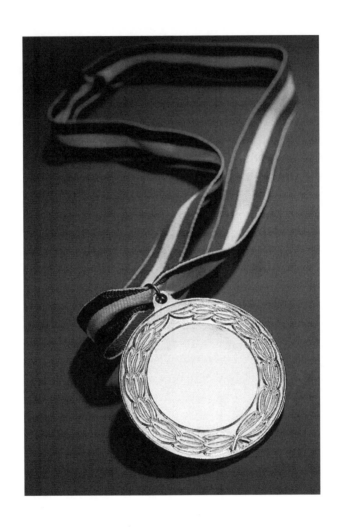

Diabetes Self Care Basics

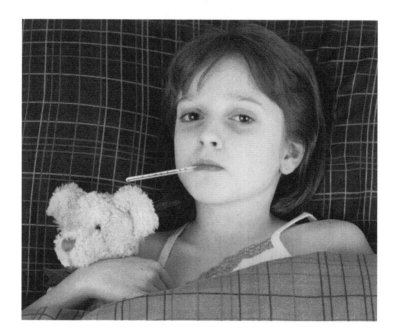

When You Are Sick

The immune system kicks into high gear to fight infections when you get a cold or flu. The fever and mediators that are released into the bloodstream during an acute illness can temporarily increase your insulin resistance -- and raise your blood sugar. Dehydration is also a risk.

If you can't eat normally or are vomiting or having diarrhea, you may temporarily drop your blood sugar. In that situation, you are at risk of low blood sugar episodes.

Monitor your blood sugar levels even more closely whenever this scenario happens. You may need to call your doctor and temporarily increase your insulin dose (if you are on insulin).

Taking plenty of fluids, more vitamin C, your multivitamins, and other antioxidants, some immune boosting herbs, and zinc lozenges may help you recover faster.

But, watch out for herb-drug interactions if you are on oral drugs that lower blood sugar. You never know if they will raise or lower your blood sugar. Call your pharmacist if you are not sure.

Regardless of the natural remedies you might try, here are some common sense tips to handle a sick day:

Call your doctor or primary health care provider if any of these happen to you:

- You feel too sick to eat normally and are unable to keep down food for more than 6 hours.

- You're having severe diarrhea.

- You lose 5 pounds or more.

- Your temperature is over 101 degrees F.

- Your blood glucose is lower than 60 mg/dL or remains over 300 mg/dL.

- You have moderate or large amounts of ketones in your urine.

- You're having trouble breathing.

- You feel sleepy or can't think clearly.

If you feel sleepy or can't think clearly, have someone call your health care provider or take you to an emergency room.

General Steps To Take At Least Once a Year

- Get a flu shot (October to mid-November).

- Get a pneumonia shot (if you've never had one).

- Get a dilated eye exam.

- Get a foot exam (including check of circulation and nerves).

- Get a kidney test.

  −Have your urine tested for microalbumin (early kidney damage from diabetes).

  −Have your blood tested for chemicals that measure your kidney function.

–Get a 24-hour urine test (if your doctor advises).

- Get your blood fats checked for:

    –Total cholesterol.

    –High-density lipoprotein (HDL).

    – Low-density lipoprotein (LDL).

    –Triglycerides

    - Vitamin D levels.

- Get a dental exam (at least twice a year).

Talk with your health care team about...

- How well you can notice symptoms when you are having a low blood glucose episode.

- How you are treating high blood glucose spikes.

- Your plans to stop tobacco use (cigarettes, cigars, pipes, smokeless tobacco), if relevant to you.

- Your feelings about having diabetes.

- Your plans for pregnancy (if a woman).

Diabetes Glossary

Use this handy glossary of diabetes related terms whenever you need to get a quick grasp of a term that your health care provider might mention.

A1C—A test that sums up how much glucose has been sticking to part of the hemoglobin (Hb) during the past 3–4 months. Hemoglobin is a substance in the red blood cells that supplies oxygen to the cells of the body.

ACE inhibitor—A type of drug used to lower blood pressure. Studies indicate that it may also help prevent or slow the progression of kidney disease in people with diabetes. ACE is an acronym for angiotensin-converting enzyme.

autoimmune process—A process where the body's immune system attacks and destroys body tissue that it mistakes for foreign matter.

beta cells—Cells that make insulin. Beta cells are found in areas of the pancreas called the Islets of Langerhans.

bladder—A hollow organ that urine drains into from the kidneys. From the bladder, urine leaves the body.

blood glucose—The main sugar that the body makes from the food we eat. Glucose is carried through the bloodstream to provide energy to all of the body's living cells. The cells cannot use glucose without the help of insulin.

blood pressure—The force of the blood against the artery walls. Two levels of blood pressure are measured: the highest, or systolic, occurs when the heart pumps blood into the blood vessels, and the lowest, or diastolic, occurs when the heart rests.

blood sugar—See blood glucose.

calluses—Thick, hardened areas of the skin, generally on the foot, caused by friction or pressure. Calluses can lead to other problems, including serious infection and even gangrene.

carbohydrate—One of three main groups of foods in the diet that provide calories and energy. (Protein and fat are the others.) Carbohydrates are mainly sugars (simple carbohydrates) and starches (complex carbohydrates, found in bread, pasta, beans) that the body breaks down into glucose.

cholesterol—A substance similar to fat that is found in the blood, muscles, liver, brain, and other body tissues. The body produces and needs some cholesterol. However, too much cholesterol can make fats stick to the walls of the arteries and cause a disease that decreases or stops circulation.

corns—A thickening of the skin of the feet or hands, usually caused by pressure against the skin.

diabetes—The short name for the disease called diabetes mellitus. Diabetes results when the body cannot use blood glucose as energy because of having too little insulin or being unable to use insulin. See also type 1 diabetes, type 2 diabetes, and gestational diabetes.

diabetes pills—Pills or capsules that are taken by mouth to help lower the blood glucose level. These pills may work for people whose bodies are still making insulin.

diabetic eye disease—A disease of the small blood vessels of the retina of the eye in people with diabetes. In this disease, the vessels swell and leak liquid into the retina, blurring the vision and sometimes leading to blindness.

diabetic ketoacidosis—High blood glucose with the presence of ketones in the urine and bloodstream, often caused by taking too little insulin or during illness.

diabetic kidney disease—Damage to the cells or blood vessels of the kidney.

diabetic nerve damage—Damage to the nerves of a person with diabetes. Nerve damage may affect the feet and hands, as well as major organs.

dialysis—A method for removing waste from the blood when the kidneys can no longer do the job.

diphtheria—An acute, contagious disease that causes fever and problems for the heart and nervous system.

EKG—A test that measures the heart's action. Also called an electrocardiogram.

flu—An infection caused by the "flu" (short for "influenza") virus. The flu is a contagious viral illness that strikes quickly and severely. Signs include high fever, chills, body aches, runny nose, sore throat, and headache.

food exchanges—A way to help people stay on special food plans by letting them replace items from one food group with items from another group.

gestational diabetes—A type of diabetes that can occur in pregnant women who have not been known to have diabetes before. Although gestational diabetes usually subsides after pregnancy, many women who've had gestational diabetes develop type 2 diabetes later in life.

gingivitis—A swelling and soreness of the gums that, without treatment, can cause serious gum problems and disease.

glucagon—A hormone that raises the blood glucose level. When someone with diabetes has a very low blood glucose level, a glucagon injection can help raise the blood glucose quickly.

glucose—A sugar in our blood and a source of energy for our bodies.

heart attack—Damage to the heart muscle caused when the blood vessels supplying the muscle are blocked, such as when the blood vessels are clogged with fats (a condition sometimes called hardening of the arteries).

HDL (or high-density lipoprotein)—A combined protein and fatlike substance. Low in cholesterol, it usually passes freely through the arteries. Sometimes called "good cholesterol."

high blood glucose—A condition that occurs in people with diabetes when their blood glucose levels are too high. Symptoms include having to urinate often, being very thirsty, and losing weight.

high blood pressure—A condition where the blood circulates through the arteries with too much force. High blood pressure tires the heart, harms the arteries, and increases the risk of heart attack, stroke, and kidney problems.

hormone—A chemical that special cells in the body release to help other cells work. For example, insulin is a hormone made in the pancreas to help the body use glucose as energy.

hyperglycemia—See high blood glucose.

hypertension—See high blood pressure.

hypoglycemia—See low blood glucose.

immunization—Sometimes called vaccination; a shot or injection that protects a person from getting an illness by making the person "immune" to it.

influenza—See flu.

inject—To force a liquid into the body with a needle and syringe.

insulin—A hormone that helps the body use blood glucose for energy. The beta cells of the pancreas make insulin. When people with diabetes can't make enough insulin, they may have to inject it from another source.

insulin-dependent diabetes—See type 1 diabetes.

ketones—Chemical substances that the body makes when it doesn't have enough insulin in the blood. When ketones build up in the body for a long time, serious illness or coma can result.

kidneys—Twin organs found in the lower part of the back. The kidneys purify the blood of all waste and harmful material. They also control the level of some helpful chemical substances in the blood.

laser surgery—Surgery that uses a strong ray of special light, called a laser, to treat damaged parts of the body. Laser surgery can help treat some diabetic eye diseases.

low blood glucose—A condition that occurs in people with diabetes when their blood glucose levels are too low. Symptoms include feeling anxious or confused, feeling numb in the arms and hands, and shaking or feeling dizzy.

LDL (or **low-density lipoprotein)**—A combined protein and fatlike substance. Rich in cholesterol, it tends to stick to the walls in the arteries. Sometimes called "bad cholesterol."

meal plan—A guide to help people get the proper amount of calories, carbohydrates, proteins, and fats in their diet. See alsofood exchanges.

microalbumin—A protein found in blood plasma and urine. The presence of microalbumin in the urine can be a sign of kidney disease.

nephropathy—See diabetic kidney disease.

neuropathy—See diabetic nerve damage.

non–insulin-dependent diabetes—See type 2 diabetes.

pancreas—An organ in the body that makes insulin so that the body can use glucose for energy. The pancreas also makes enzymes that help the body digest food.

periodontitis—A gum disease in which the gums shrink away from the teeth. Without treatment, it can lead to tooth loss.

plaque—A film of mucus that traps bacteria on the surface of the teeth. Plaque can be removed with daily brushing and flossing of teeth.

pumice stone—A special foot care tool used to gently file calluses as instructed by your health care team.

retinopathy—See diabetic eye disease.

risk factors—Traits that make it more likely that a person will get an illness. For example, a risk factor for getting type 2 diabetes is having a family history of diabetes.

self-monitoring blood glucose—A way for people with diabetes to find out how much glucose is in their blood. A drop of blood from the fingertip is placed on a special coated strip of paper that "reads" (often through an electronic meter) the amount of glucose in the blood.

stroke—Damage to a part of the brain that happens when the blood vessels supplying that part are blocked, such as when the blood vessels are clogged with fats (a condition sometimes called hardening of the arteries).

support group—A group of people who share a similar problem or concern. The people in the group help one another by sharing experiences, knowledge, and information.

type 1 diabetes—A condition in which the pancreas makes so little insulin that the body can't use blood glucose as energy. Type 1 diabetes most often occurs in people younger than age 30 and must be controlled with daily insulin injections.

type 2 diabetes—A condition in which the body either makes too little insulin or can't use the insulin it makes to use blood glucose as energy. Type 2 diabetes most often occurs in people older than age 40 and can often be controlled through meal plans and physical activity plans. Some people with type 2 diabetes have to take diabetes pills by mouth and/or insulin by injection.

ulcer —A break or deep sore in the skin. Germs can enter an ulcer and may be hard to heal.

urea—One of the chief waste products of the body. When the body breaks down food, it uses what it needs and throws the rest away as waste. The kidneys flush the waste from the body in the form of urea, which is in the urine.

vaccination—A shot given to protect against a disease.

vagina—A canal in females from the external genitalia (vulva) to the cervix of the uterus.

162

vitrectomy—An operation to remove the blood that sometimes collects at the back of the eyes when a person has eye disease.

yeast infection —A vaginal infection that is usually caused by a fungus. Women who have this infection may feel itching, burning when urinating, and pain, and some women have a vaginal discharge. Yeast infections occur more frequently in women with diabetes.

Public Domain Source:
http://www.cdc.gov/diabetes/pubs/tcyd/appendix.htm

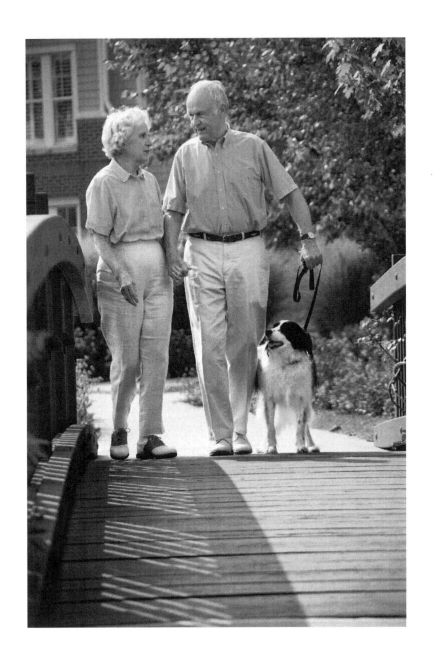

Diabetes Resources

General Information on Diabetes

U.S. National Library of Medicine:

www.ncbi.nlm.nih.gov/pubmedhealth/PMH0002194

American Diabetes Association:

www.diabetes.org

Juvenile Diabetes Research Foundation:

www.jdrf.org

U.S. Centers for Disease Control & Prevention:

www.cdc.gov/diabetes

News and Updates on Natural Ways to Lower Blood Sugar:

www.HighBloodSugarSolution.com

Tools for Controlling Your Blood Sugar

No Calorie, Low Carb Shirataki Noodles:

www.highbloodsugarsolution.com/shirataki-noodles

Food Scale with Calorie, Protein, Carbohydrate, Fat, and Glycemic Index Read-outs:

www.highbloodsugarsolution.com/304/digital-food-scales-in-diabetes/

Striiv Personal Trainer in a Pocket Device:

www.howtosticktoadiet.org/28/weight-loss-motivation-tip-use-biofeedback/

Get Your Free Quick Start Resource Kit to Lower Blood Sugar Naturally

www.DefyingDiabetesPlan.com

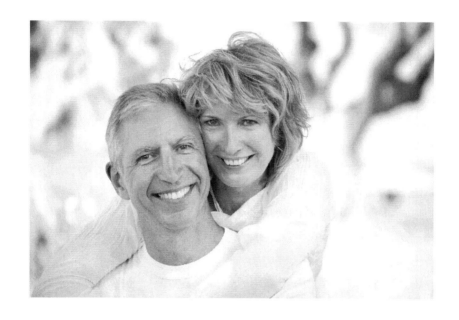

Printed in Great Britain
by Amazon.co.uk, Ltd.,
Marston Gate.